Wisdom
of
the East

Stories of
Compassion,
Inspiration,
and Love

Wisdom
of
the East

Stories of
Compassion,
Inspiration,
and Love

COLLECTED AND EDITED BY
SUSAN SUNTREE

Foreword by His Holiness
the Fourteenth Dalai Lama

Contemporary Books

Chicago New York San Francisco Lisbon London Madrid Mexico City
Milan New Delhi San Juan Seoul Singapore Sydney Toronto

Library of Congress Cataloging-in-Publication Data

Wisdom from the East : stories of compassion, inspiration, and love / collected and
edited by Susan Suntree.
    p. cm.
ISBN 0-7373-0584-3 (alk. paper)
1. Spiritual life. I. Suntree, Susan.
BL624 .W58 2001
291.4'4--dc21   2001047049

Contemporary Books

A Division of The McGraw·Hill Companies

1 2 3 4 5 6 7 8 9 0   LBM/LBM   0 9 8 7 6 5 4 3 2 1

ISBN 0-7373-0584-3

This book was set in ITC Legacy Serif and designed by Laurie Young
Printed and bound by Lake Book Manufacturing

Cover design by Laurie Young
Cover illustration by Melissa McGill

McGraw-Hill books are available at special quantity discounts to use as premiums and sales
promotions, or for use in corporate training programs. For more information, please write to
the Director of Special Sales, Professional Publishing, McGraw-Hill, Two Penn Plaza, New
York, NY 10121-2298. Or contact your local bookstore.

This book is printed on recycled, acid-free paper.

CONTENTS

FOREWORD by His Holiness the Fourteenth Dalai Lama   *xi*

ACKNOWLEDGMENTS   *xv*

INTRODUCTION   *xvii*

MICHAEL J. TAMURA   *3*
Seeking First That Which Gives Everything

MELODY ERMACHILD CHAVIS   *9*
Going to Prison

ROBERT AITKEN   *17*
Carvers

AUTUMN JACOBSEN   *21*
Slowly It Is Coming

MERLE PENDELL   *29*
The Red-Hot Iron Ball

WAHEED SIDDIQEE   *33*
The Wisdom of Mothers, Poets, and Saints

CONTENTS

SOGYAL RINPOCHE *39*
Mindfulness in Everyday Life

E. H. RICK JAROW *43*
Sripada

vi

WENDY EGYOKU NAKAO *51*
Come and See

JOHN ADAMS *57*
Lost in Movement, Found in Stillness

NORMAN FISCHER *63*
My Mother

GESHE TSULTIM GYELTSEN *69*
The Buddha's Great Heart

FORD ROOSEVELT *75*
Buddhism and the Roosevelt Legacy

CHRISTOPHER TITMUSS *81*
Awareness: Springboard for Meditation and Politics

JILL ANSELL *89*
Asanga and the B Yard

DIANE RIZZETTO *95*
Hide and Seek

CAROL LEM *101*
Suizen: Blowing Meditation

MASAKAZU YOSHIZAWA *109*
My Music, My Destiny

ROBERT NICHOLS *115*
Life As a Work of Art

BABA HARI DASS *121*
God Is Peace

Contents

BOB COHEN   *127*
Saint or Sinner?

MATTHIEU RICARD   *133*
The Life of Shabkar

CHERI CLAMPETT   *139*
A Knowing Beyond Words

THICH NHAT HANH   *145*
The Peace of the Divine Reality

BO LOZOFF   *153*
The Samurai and the Zen Master

JACQUIE BELLON   *157*
You're Preapproved: Accept Today

SUSAN MOON   *163*
Who Isn't Busy?

PEMA CHÖDRÖN   *173*
Finding Our Own True Nature

DALE PENDELL   *181*
Sauntering with Lao–tzu

MICHAEL BARNARD   *187*
The Infinite Well

BARBARA J. HODGSON   *193*
Being Truly Home

SURINDER MANN   *201*
The Front Room

JOKO BECK   *205*
The Key

CYNTHIA LESTER   *211*
Death, Not Death

CONTENTS

GRACE BRUMETT   *215*
Gone Beyond: A Question of Letting Go

GRAHAM M. SCHWEIG   *223*
Beauty Captures Devotee and Divinity

viii   **KEVIN KREIGER**   *231*
Into the Deep

ANDREW HARVEY   *237*
Honor the Sacred Feminine

MICHAEL ATTIE   *245*
Memoirs of a Lingerie Monk

HER EMINENCE SAKYA DAGMO KUSHO   *251*
Homage to Tara

BARBARA PENN   *257*
Just This

JIM RYAN   *263*
A New View of Time

MARK ROBERT WALDMAN   *267*
I Was a Jewish Atheistic Ministerial Counselor with a Buddhist Practice Who
Prayed to God, Went with the Taoist Flow, Embraced Confucian Morals, and
Frolicked with a Hindu Goddess or Two

SHIVA REA   *271*
Life As Offering

MATTHEW COLEMAN   *277*
Composting Light

SHINZEN YOUNG   *281*
O Night That Unites: A Personal Appreciation of St. John of the Cross

PHYLLIS WATTS   *287*
The Soft Underbelly of Life

Contents

SUSAN SUNTREE   *293*
The Green Bean *Sutra*

GARY SNYDER   *299*
Grace

MATTHIEU RICARD   *305*
The Practice of Compassion

BO LOZOFF   *309*
Ted

APPENDIX A
Universal Declaration of Human Rights   *313*

PERMISSIONS   *321*

ABOUT THE EDITOR   *325*

INDEX   *327*

FOREWORD

When I meet people in different parts of the world, I am always reminded that we are all basically alike: we are all human beings. Maybe we wear different clothes, our skin is of a different color, or we speak different languages. These are only superficial differences. Basically, we are the same human beings. That is what makes it possible for us to understand each other and to develop friendship and closeness.

Let me share with you a short prayer, which gives me great inspiration in my own quest to be of benefit to others:

> *May I become at all times, both now and forever*
> *A protector for those without protection*
> *A guide for those who have lost their way*
> *A ship for those with oceans to cross*
> *A bridge for those with rivers to cross*
> *A sanctuary for those in danger*
> *A lamp for those without light*
> *A place of refuge for those who lack shelter*
> *And a servant to all in need.*

The core of this advice is to make your life as meaningful as possible. There is nothing mysterious about it. It consists of nothing more than acting out of concern for others. And provided you undertake this practice sincerely and with persistence, you will gradually be able to reorder your habits and attitudes so that you think less about your own narrow concerns and more about the concerns of others. In doing so, you will find that you enjoy peace and happiness yourself.

Relinquish your envy; let go your desire to triumph over others. Instead, try to benefit them. With kindness, courage, and confidence that in doing so you are sure to meet with success, welcome others with a smile. Be straightforward. And try to be impartial. Treat everyone as if they were close friends. I say this as a human being: one who, like yourself, wishes to be happy and not miserable.

If you cannot, for whatever reason, be of help to others, at least don't harm them. Consider yourself a tourist. Think of the world as it is seen from space, so small and insignificant yet so beautiful. Is there really anything to be gained from harming others during our stay here? Is it not preferable, and more reasonable, to relax and enjoy ourselves quietly, just as if we were visiting a different neighborhood? If in the midst of your enjoyment of the world you have a moment, try to help, in however small a way, those who are downtrodden and those who, for whatever reason, cannot or do not help themselves. Try not to turn away from those whose appearance is disturbing, from the ragged and unwell. Try never to think of them as inferior to yourself. If you can, try not even to think of yourself as better than the humblest beggar, for we will all look the same in the grave.

Because we all share this small planet Earth, we have to learn to live in harmony and peace with each other and with nature. That is not just a dream but a necessity. We are dependent on each other in so many ways that we can no longer live in isolated communities and ignore what is happening outside those communities. We need to help each other when we have difficulties, and we must share the good fortune that we enjoy.

I would also like to mention here the plight and aspirations of the people of Tibet. As a free spokesman for my fellow countrymen and women, I feel it is my duty to speak out on their behalf. But I do so not with a feeling of anger or hatred toward those who are responsible for the immense suffering of our people and the destruction of our land, homes, and culture. I make a distinction between the action and its perpetrator. Moreover, the Chinese, too, are human beings who struggle to find happiness and deserve our compassion. I do so simply to draw attention to the sad situation in my country today and to the aspirations of my people, because in our struggle for freedom, truth is the only weapon we possess.

We Tibetans also hope to contribute to the development of a more peaceful, more humane, and more beautiful world. A future free Tibet will seek to help those in need throughout the world, to protect nature, and to promote peace. I believe that the Tibetan ability to combine spiritual qualities with a realistic and practical attitude enables us to make a special contribution, in however modest a way.

Finally, let me conclude with another verse from the great eighth-century Indian Buddhist master, Shantideva:

> *For as long as space endures,*
> *And for as long as living beings remain,*
> *Until then may I, too, abide*
> *To dispel the misery of the world.*

> —HIS HOLINESS THE FOURTEENTH DALAI LAMA
> November 6, 2000

ACKNOWLEDGMENTS

Creating *Wisdom of the East: Stories of Compassion, Inspiration, and Love* has been a thoroughly collaborative task, bringing together the insights, words, and labor of many people. Mark Waldman, the editor of the New Vision series in which this book appears, has offered consistent support. He generously shared with me his wealth of experience editing anthologies, and he did this with his unique good humor, cooking skills, and steadiness of purpose. Miriyam Glazer, who edited *Dancing on the Edge of the World: Jewish Stories of Faith, Inspiration, and Love*, another book in this series, suggested to Mark that I edit this volume. Her confidence inspired my work from its initiation to its completion. Shaping a collection that includes fifty authors from around the world is an adventure that requires word processing and organizational skills *par excellence*. Without the acumen and dedication of my assistant, Lola Terrell, compiling and editing this anthology may well have devolved into chaos without the regenerative powers of wisdom and compassion! Another person who has been essential to this project is Califia Suntree, my editorial assistant. Her skill is like a sculptor's: she sees the spirit and intent of a piece and hones the words until they are unmistakably clear.

Many people guided me to the contributors represented in this collection. I am especially grateful to Jill Ansell, James Bailey, Giza Braun, Valerie

Fowler, Ruth Ghio, Kathy Gronau, Joni Harlan, the Buddhist Peace Fellowship Office, Barbara Hodgson, Cynthia Lester, and Mary Wright. Paul and Elina O'Lague provided abundant technical and moral support. Two groups of women have affirmed, critiqued, and sustained me and my work as a writer: I offer my heartfelt thanks and appreciation to the members of Writers' Circle (Deborah Bogen, Chris Ferris, Deirdre Gainer, Mary Jansen, Bronwen Sennish, and Zoey Zimmerman) and to the Women's Lunch Group (Susan Chehak, Jo Giese, Yasmin Kafai, Rae Lewis, Jo Ann Matyas, Luchita Mullican, Virginia Mullin, Maria Munroe, Doreen Nelson, Nancy Nimoy, Amanda Pope, Judith Searle, Carolyn See, and Janet Sternburg). I offer my heartfelt thanks, also, to John Runnette for his unflagging kindness, especially during the weeks spent finishing this project.

Most significantly, I am indebted to the authors, whose generous stories made my work a joy.

INTRODUCTION

Prison yards, caves, and Tibetan highland monasteries; sensual celebrations of beauty in classical Hindu poetry; the strife-ravaged Middle East; the deathbed of a loved one; intimate moments when the world is experienced whole even if only for a few moments. The authors in this anthology take us to the core of trouble and suffering, beauty and joy. Their stories show us the power of compassion to demonstrate our innate kinship with the world, and show us how to exchange the burden of the lonely, isolated self for the magnificent container that is all of life.

The word *compassion* is derived from the fusion of two Latin words: *com* meaning "together with," and *pati,* meaning "suffering." So compassion means to "suffer together," a perception that can transform self-interest or greed. In Siberia and Central Asia, the practice of traditional shamanism is rooted in a concept of the universe as a totality in which all its members are permeable. Barriers between form and energy and between nature and humanity dissolve in the shaman's ecstatic vision. This notion is central to the act of compassion. As the fourteenth-century Christian mystic Meister Eckhart observed, "The other is no other than myself."

The works assembled here offer an intimate glimpse of how wisdom and compassion are actually lived. In Gary Snyder's story, "Grace," saying thank you before eating a meal is as profound a moment as any we might ever encounter, connecting us to the life-in-death that is at the core of our universe. While some authors, such as Dale Pendell, write about the pleasures of reading classical texts, for Grace Brumett and Wendy Egyoku Nakao they are guides through loss and grief. Some writers observe how the text is experience itself: a posture that teaches yoga, a bamboo flute that teaches the aspiring shakuhachi musician. Robert Aitken links insights from his practice as a Zen teacher with lines from the poetry of John Donne. Sustaining and practical, these stories offer the reader bridges connecting East and West and day-to-day life with revelatory moments of extraordinary pleasure or pain.

British Vipassana teacher and activist Christopher Titmuss and anti–death penalty activist and writer Melody Ermachild Chavis show us how they remain steady and free to love as various kinds of prison doors slam shut behind them. Thich Nhat Hanh shares a poem written by a long-forgotten writer from the Vietnam War era. French photojournalist and monk Matthieu Ricard recounts the lives of two Tibetan teachers whose intense struggles and dedication provide role models for how to face inevitable personal and political dilemmas. Finally, Bo Lozoff's friend and teacher, a "hillbilly, ex-con truck driver" named Ted, takes us straight to the heart of the matter.

This anthology abounds with insights into how compassion inextricably relates us to everyone and everything, thus making us all into activists, or, as Andrew Harvey writes, "revolutionaries of love." In a world replete with violence and seemingly overwhelmed by the greed that pumps the global economy, the need for compassion resides at the forefront of many people's minds. Ford Roosevelt, the grandson of Eleanor and Franklin D. Roosevelt, describes his fateful meeting with the executive director of Amnesty International who reminds him that his grandmother chaired the committee that wrote the International Declaration of Human Rights. When he later meets His Holiness the Fourteenth Dalai Lama, Roosevelt connects his practice of Tibetan Buddhism to his commitment to disseminating this inspiring document. In honor of His Holiness and as encouragement for us all, I include the complete text of the Declaration in Appendix A.

As an environmental activist, it is easy for me to feel immeasurably discouraged as the landscape deteriorates and wildlife habitat disappears. The number of campaigns lost outweighs those I count as won, and sometimes I feel invisible when speaking out about the injustice of decimating a wetland or directing pollution into poor neighborhoods. So, I am grateful for the models of activism rooted in practical compassion described in several selections. They urge me to actually, rather than conceptually, reside in the web of life. I see how the work of compassionate people radiates into society, countering the dominant preoccupation with self-aggrandizement. Such people are well represented in this collection.

Editing *Wisdom of the East* has allowed me to spend time with each author's experience of wisdom, compassion, inspiration, and love. When I first began, I simply asked contributors to respond to a favorite story or poem from their spiritual tradition. I wanted them to write about how these words shaped or changed their lives, or how they helped them through trying circumstances or just an ordinary day. Though the focus of this book is Asian-based spiritual paths, I discovered that the world's religions mingle fruitfully in these teachers and practitioners. Resonating at the core of each story is an understanding that everything is interrelated—squash blossoms, barbed wire fences, the paper of this book.

Readers will also find here an extraordinary fount of quotations—those that have privately inspired some of the most influential teachers of our day as well as devoted practitioners. These lines are drawn from Buddhist, Taoist, Sikh, Hindu, Islamic, and Christian sources. To maintain the unique expression of the authors, I have retained their spelling of ancient Asian languages such as Pali, the language used during Buddha's life, and Sanskrit, the language used to record early Buddhist and Hindu scriptures. Whether these quotations confront or comfort us, they are meant to disturb our fixed sense of ourselves. Vibrant with the authors' sincerity and commitment, they guide us on a marvelous adventure of the heart where many worlds meet and find their commonality.

Seek ye first that which gives you everything
and everything shall be given to you.

BHAGAVAD GITA

MICHAEL J. TAMURA

Seeking First That Which Gives Everything

"IT'S ALL RIGHT, LITTLE ONE. IT'S GOING TO BE ALL RIGHT."

A mixture of dread that I have done something horribly wrong, hope that everything will turn out all right, and the simple love of life churned with urgency in my chest.

"I'm just going to pick you up. I don't think it's going to hurt too much more. Okay?"

Deep sobs erupted from within me as I fitfully reached down to the concrete pavement. Gingerly, I picked up the two writhing halves of the large earthworm. All I could imagine was what it would feel like to be suddenly broken in half. My delight and excitement at finding a new set of chin-up bars to play on spilled out of me onto the pavement in large, vision-blurring droplets. I realized that I had accidentally stepped on the worm and split the poor creature in two. I was five years old.

I held the worm's broken pieces squirming in agony in my hands. I ran home with them from my friend's backyard as fast as my legs could move. Wiping the warm, salty tears streaming down my cheeks, I rummaged through drawers and cabinets looking for something—anything— I could use to put the worm back together.

I finally found a roll of Scotch tape and some Kleenex. I cut and carefully folded a tiny piece of the tissue, enough to go once around the belly of the earthworm. Then, I laid the piece of Kleenex on a strip of tape so that a small portion of it remained uncovered at one end. Ever so gently, I wrapped the makeshift bandage around the cut while I held the two parts of the worm together. Miraculously, the creature cooperated, staying still.

"Be very still, little one. I know you'll be okay soon. I know this must hurt very bad, but you'll be all right soon. I promise!" I spoke to it and placed it in a shoebox.

No one had taught me about prayer as such, but somehow I knew to pray. I prayed to an unseen, but not an unfelt, Presence. I asked that this worm be made whole again, that it would be relieved of its suffering. I just knew that if I asked with all my heart, my wish would be granted.

Whoever answers prayers didn't fail me. The worm grew visibly stronger each day. By the third day, I took the bandage off. The worm was whole and I felt that I had made a new friend. I took it back to my friend's backyard and let it wiggle out of the shoebox to freedom.

Looking back at that innocent wisdom of my childhood, I find the beginning of my life as a spiritual healer and teacher. The heart of wisdom is truly the wisdom of the heart. All healing begins—and ends—with love. This particular love story comes from Japan.

I was born in the land of the rising sun, the birthplace of the *samurai* and home to *bushido,* the way of the warrior. I came into this world eight years after the two *pikari* (intense flashes) of light that forever changed the way humanity looks at war and ushered in a new consciousness that everything is energy.

My mother was a native-born Japanese; in her early teens she worked in a factory recycling ordnance for the war effort. My father-to-be was *nisei* (second-generation Japanese American), interned in the United States during the war in which his father and a younger sister perished in Hiroshima. Genetically speaking, I am "made in Japan" through and through, although I was born an American citizen.

I grew up in Tokyo. At home I spoke Japanese and at school on the American base I spoke English. I had Japanese friends in my neighborhood and American friends at the base. I ate good old American cafeteria food at school while feasting on Japanese delicacies at home. I always loved the tap-estry of my life, woven from diverse threads of culture and race.

Perhaps it was the occasional references to the *kami-sama* (divine spirits) that I heard from my mother, grandmother, other relatives, and my nannies that first validated what I intuitively knew: There was some unseen Spirit that created things of the world and with whom we could communicate.

5

On rainy days we made special dolls from square pieces of colored tis-sue. We would ball up a small amount of tissue in the center of the colored square and tie a thread around it to make a round head with a trailing rain-coat. We'd make several of them and hang them from the eaves. They were our messages to the spirits to stop the rain and bring out the sunshine.

At other times, I remember making *origami* (intricately folded colored paper) cranes for blessings of prosperity and well-being, both for ourselves and others. Communicating with the spirits and seeking their help were not religious rituals for me. They were real, practical, and readily accessible. Though the Japan I grew up in was rapidly industrializing and gravitating toward Western ways, the land itself still held the Shinto spirit of honoring divinity in nature. Divinity was natural. Perhaps this made it easier for me to seek an inner source as I did in my early healing experiences. I knew what I asked for would be granted.

I left home when I was sixteen years old and came to live in the United States. Within a year, I began my spiritual search in earnest. I didn't know what it was I was looking for. All I knew was that I had to find it. If there was a door I tried to open it: martial arts, yoga, meditation, mysticism, Chinese medicine, Indian scriptures. Somewhere in my teenage spiritual foraging, what I had always felt within myself was incarnated. It took the form of a quote from Krishna:

"Seek ye first that which gives you everything and everything shall be given to you."

I knew that was what I had always sought and what I was seeking then. I was not seeking some omnipotent god, but the experience of that which gave me everything. I was seeking that Spirit I knew and had communicated with as a child. It was that which gave wholeness back to the earthworm.

This beautiful passage from the *Bhagavad Gita* brought to my conscious awareness the truth that has surfaced time and again in my life. Much later, I discovered that another avatar, Jesus Christ, had spoken almost the very same words: "Seek ye first the kingdom of God and all else shall be added unto you." When One who embodies Divinity tells you what to seek first, wouldn't it be foolish to do otherwise?

6

Today, each morning before pursuing any activity or any goal, I first turn my awareness to that which gives me everything. After all, if we desire water, we won't hold the empty bucket turned away from the faucet. Only when we turn toward the faucet and hold our bucket beneath it, can we have our fill of water. We must turn our awareness inward, toward our spiritual faucet.

We are enjoying an era of unparalleled technological advances that help us live more comfortable and productive lives. Yet, we cannot afford to become complacent and allow the flood of material progress to extinguish the fire within our hearts. More than ever we need to turn our consciousness to the purpose of life itself.

The atom bomb was a human invention. But the power it unleashed was all God's. Hiroshima demonstrated mankind's spiritual inadequacy to wield the inconceivable power contained in every atom of existence. It put the world, for the first time, under the threat of annihilation by humanity itself. Our arrogance was humbled into an awareness of how much we must still learn and grow.

Within every tragedy is buried the seed of a greater healing. Our task is to find this seed, plant it in our hearts, and nourish it with the water of Spirit that gives life. To find this seed we must first seek that which gives us everything.

Michael J. Tamura, a spiritual teacher, healer, and clairvoyant, lives in Colorado with his wife, Raphaelle, who is also a healer and teacher, and his two sons. His Web site is www.michaeltamura.com.

Don't worry about whether you like it or don't like it.
Just do it, and your life will blossom.

KATAGIRI ROSHI

◈

MELODY ERMACHILD CHAVIS

Going to Prison

I HAVE HAD A LONG RELATIONSHIP WITH SAN QUENTIN PRISON.

For twenty years now I've worked as a private investigator, helping to defend people on death row. Several times a month I drive to the windy prison parking lot beside a little cove on San Francisco Bay and walk up the hill to the gate. Various correctional officers buzz me through locked doors; scan my shoes, jacket, and legal files through two metal detectors; and stamp my hand with yellow fluorescent ink. By now I've worked at San Quentin longer than most of the officers, but because I don't wear a uniform, and I work for the rights of prisoners, some officers treat me as if I don't belong there.

Recently, a pretty young blond officer I'd never seen before answered my pleasant "good morning" with a bark. "Now listen up to what I'm going to tell you," she commanded. "I'm only going to say this once. Your visit will be in cell A-1." I could feel my smile fade away as I said, "Thank you," and retrieved my license that she had slapped down on the desk.

I always carry a little date book into the prison to mark my future appointments with my clients. Scribbled inside the back cover is something a Zen teacher said. Sometimes while I'm waiting in line at the metal detector I remember to flip that page open and read it to myself:

Don't worry about whether you like it or don't like it.
Just do it, and your life will blossom.

KATAGIRI ROSHI

These two sentences wake me up to the fact that my life doesn't stop
when I go to prison, and it doesn't start again when I get out. This is my
life, right now. Katagiri Roshi's words remind me that clinging to prefer-
ences will only limit my experience.

I never knew Katagiri Roshi. He was a Zen priest who came from
Japan to teach in America, and he died some years ago. Not far from San
Quentin, at Green Gulch Zen monastery, a carved white stone high on a
grassy hill commemorates his life. I became a student of this teacher I never
met when I read this quote and copied it into my date book. Every January
since, in each fresh book, I've written it again. Carried into the prison, this
little bit of wisdom seems so valuable, it feels like contraband.

But it's hard not to think about what I like and don't like. In fact,
sometimes I hate San Quentin and what happens inside it so much, I want
to show that gate my back and never enter it again. Sometimes the block-
long sidewalk that leads along the bay to the second set of walls and metal
detectors seems like a steep uphill mile. I wonder why I'm taking myself to
prison again. Sometimes, when my spirits sink as I walk under the watchful
eyes in the gun towers, I think of Sammy, a death row prisoner who was
killed in San Quentin.

He was not my client, and I did not know him. I would never have
known how he died, except that my friend Jarvis, also a prisoner on death
row, witnessed it, looking down the tier with his tiny shard of mirror.
Sammy was one of San Quentin's fully psychotic prisoners. Jarvis said that
for a long time before his death, Sammy was unable to clean himself or his
cell; he raved day and night and slept only for short periods. Sammy barely
ate because he was afraid his food was poisoned, and he refused to come
out of his cell for exercise or showers.

Then a near-miracle happened. Sammy's lawyers won his appeal. He
was ordered transferred from death row back to the jail in the county he

had come from, to await a new trial. But Sammy did not understand. When the day came for Sammy to get on the prison bus, he couldn't comprehend why people wanted him to walk out of his cell, and he refused. He cowered in the back of the cell, shaking his head and talking to himself.

So the authorities assigned an extraction team—half a dozen or so unlucky officers—to take Sammy out of his cell by force. Burly men, they wear boots, helmets, gloves, protective gas masks, and all-white jump suits. Jarvis, trying to describe them, said they look like members of some space-age Ku Klux Klan. When Sammy saw them in front of his cell, he crawled under his mattress and screamed. The officers then sprayed canisters of pepper spray into Sammy's cell to subdue him. Hoping he would run out to get away from the spray, the officers tried to open the wire mesh door to the cell. But Sammy had woven strips of torn blanket in and out of the mesh, tying the door tightly to the front wall of the cell. It took the officers a long time to send for a saw and to tear away the tough fabric. When they finally got the door open, Sammy was unconscious.

The other prisoners were shouting at the officers to help him. The prisoners wanted the officers to wheel Sammy, by now lying on a gurney, into the shower on the tier and wash the pepper spray off him. Instead, they pushed him out of the security-housing unit, and the door slammed shut behind them.

It was some time before Jarvis and the other anxious prisoners heard, from other officers and prisoners, that they had taken Sammy to the prison infirmary and left him there without alerting anyone. The medical staff found him on the gurney half an hour later—dead. Jarvis and I have no way of knowing the truth of this account. All we know is that Sammy died like a homeless old man—with only a few to mourn him, and nobody who can do much of anything about it. "They gave Sammy the gas chamber," Jarvis said.

If I do not get wrapped up in how much I dislike what was done to Sammy, I have a better chance of working effectively to tell people about such abuses and to prevent them. Katagiri Roshi is telling me to get out of my own way. I've forgotten now where I read Katagiri Roshi's advice. I think that Katagiri was referring to meditation. Perhaps he was answering a student who asked about the pain of sitting still for a long time.

"Don't worry," Katagiri said. Don't worry about whether your leg is hurting. Don't worry about your mind filling up with things you have to do. Just sit. Just keep bringing your mind back to your breath. Just bring your body back to your cushion. Just keep bringing yourself back here to your life, right now. Just sit in the middle of everything, even in the middle of San Quentin, as Jarvis does when he meditates sitting on a folded blanket in his cell. I remember Katagiri's words and I think, "Just keep walking into this prison. Just put one foot in front of the other and enter the gate."

If I just—only—walk through the gate, I am suddenly free to be there. If I'm not busy hating San Quentin, I can notice the whitecaps blowing on the bay against its walls and remember that these hours inside are precious. I have too many clients, appointments are hard to get, and for some, I'm the only visitor who ever comes. An hour to talk together really matters to both of us. Both of us can learn.

It's harder for me to feel like my time with correctional officers is equally precious. I get to know my clients fairly well, but nearly everything about the officers—their home lives, thoughts, and feelings—is a mystery. There are many officers who seem kind, even some who say, "Are you seeing Jarvis today? Say hi to him for me." But in the back of my mind is always the question: Which officers were behind those gas masks when Sammy was killed? Who are the men and women—their identities kept a close secret—who volunteer to carry out the executions?

There is one older officer, a short white man who never smiles, who sometimes guards the visiting area. With a scowl, he points me toward the legal visiting booth, a dimly lit, closetlike space where I sit on a hard plastic chair opposite my client and talk to him through a window of metal mesh. Over the years, I've had my problems with that officer, and I guess he would say he's had problems with me. Once, he caught me trying to shove a candy bar through the narrow port at the bottom of the wire mesh. The ports are supposed to be used for passing legal papers, not chocolate. The grouchy officer opened the door behind me as I was trying to push a too-fat

Snickers bar under the metal. The chocolate had peeled back, the caramel was all over my fingers and the bar was stuck halfway between the prisoner and me.

I didn't feel very guilty. After all, I hadn't smuggled the candy in—I'd bought it at the prison's own vending machine. I'm allowed to buy candy and soda for most of my death row clients, with whom I have "contact visits." But it's against the rules to pass food to those in the high-security housing unit—like Jarvis—who must visit from behind the mesh.

The guard terminated my visit and wrote an order that for the next several months I had to interview my high-security clients only on the phone, with a solid pane of glass between us. Holding a phone for hours on end gave me an aching elbow and neck, and I felt sorely punished. I had a tiny taste of the arbitrary and petty power held over the lives of my clients. I learned my lesson, and my short-lived crime spree at San Quentin was over.

One day a couple of years later, I was in one of those grim booths visiting with Jarvis, and we were laughing a lot. Jarvis loves visits, and he enjoys them as if we were sharing a sunny day at the beach. Jarvis really knows what it means to stop worrying about whether he likes San Quentin or not. He says that the second he starts thinking about wanting to get out of there, he starts doing really hard time. That day, I was entertaining him with tales of funny things my little grandchildren do and say. And he was telling me all about the latest cute doings of his nephews and nieces. As I emerged smiling from the booth, walking backwards and waving at Jarvis, who was being handcuffed for his trip back to his cell, I nearly bumped into that same grumpy guard. In a scathing tone he inquired, "Did you *enjoy* your visit?" Meaning, I should not be having a good time with a client on death row; I should be *working*, not laughing.

I was struck dumb by his question for a second, and I mumbled, with a sheepish smile, "I guess so." Then I added, defensively, "I mean, I'm working."

The officer and I both had to wait for the gate to be buzzed open. I looked at him, standing stiffly, cinched by his thick leather belt, the ring of heavy keys hanging off it. He looked so miserably locked up: "Locked up, locked down, locked in, locked out," I thought, gazing at him. Right then, I stopped disliking him. The tension of standing near him eased out of my body. "Do you know," I ventured, "this year is my twentieth year in this job. I decided quite a while ago that I might as well try to enjoy it. I hope you can enjoy your time here, at least a little." I really meant it, and he could tell. He looked surprised for a second. Then he shook his head and shoulders and made a sort of "Hrumpf!" sound in reply, like a bird ruffling its feathers. The old gate began to move noisily on its track, and, frowning again, he shoved through it ahead of me.

He and I have seen each other many times since then, and we treat each other now with a kind of distant respect. Something happened that day by the gate that changed the resentment between us. When Katagiri Roshi said that my life will blossom if I stop worrying about whether I like things or not, he didn't mean that San Quentin would suddenly fill up with flowers instead of pain. But the more I can give up liking or disliking the place, the more blooms I will find there, inside of me and out.

Melody Ermachild Chavis works as a private investigator on death penalty cases and as a community volunteer. She is the author of *Altars in the Street: A Neighborhood Fights to Survive* (1997) and is a *Sierra* essay contest winner.

Carvers do not faces make,
But that away, which hid them there, do take.

JOHN DONNE, "THE CROSSE"

✦

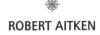

ROBERT AITKEN

Carvers

I FOUND DONNE'S METAPHOR IN R. H. BLYTH'S *Zen in English Literature and Oriental Classics* when I was twenty-six years old, interned in Japan during World War II. Here is the context:

> *Then you are to yourself a Crucifixe.*
> *As perchance, Carvers do not faces make,*
> *But that away, which hid them there, do take;*
> *Let crosses, soe, take what hid Christ in thee,*
> *And be his image, or not his, but hee.*

As someone not oriented toward religion at the time, the Carvers metaphor was the nut of the poem for me. Early seventeenth-century English vocabulary and construction veiled the meaning at first. It took me a while to understand that carvers are sculptors, and then to understand what all sculptors know, that the image is hidden in the uncarved log or marble. As Thoreau says, we carve our faces from the raw stuff with which we are born.

Another good while passed before I could take in the other lines and appreciate Donne's complete meaning, a profound restatement of the injunction of Jesus, "Take up thy cross and follow me." Our crosses empower us to dislodge the stuff that hides the Christ that is our true being.

I think of the metaphor occasionally in my Zen practice—chiseling and sandpapering my face—and in my teaching—offering tools for students to do likewise. However, sins are the cross of Christians, and the burden of Zen Buddhists can be described as the poisons of greed, hatred, and ignorance. Not the same freight in words, and certainly not in fact.

18
Still, freed of sectarian limitations, the metaphor is very helpful. I am a greedy, hateful, and ignorant fellow. That is my nature, my self, and I work hard on the primordial path of inclusive wisdom that our ancestors clarified. My students work hard on that path, too. Gradually, perhaps with sudden openings, the troublesome self drops away and something emerges authentically me, or authentically others in their uniqueness and variety. Not as the Christ, not as the Buddha, not as the "original face," but, say, as a rainbow, the moon, or a thrush.

"Who hears that thrush?" With that question there might be a peak experience, but the work continues thereafter.

Robert Aitken is the retired master of the Honolulu Diamond Sangha, a Zen Buddhist society, now living on the Big Island of Hawaii.

Do your practice, all is coming.

SRI K. PATTABHI JOIS

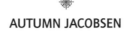

AUTUMN JACOBSEN

Slowly It Is Coming

I.

SOME CALL ME A YOGI-EVANGELIST. I HAVE TRIED TO ARGUE WITH THIS TITLE, BUT I gave up and admit that perhaps I am. I am not out to convert anyone into a yogi, but I have a hard time staying quiet about yoga's power. I practice Ashtanga Vinyasa yoga, a complex system of six series of *asanas* (postures). The guru of Ashtanga Vinyasa yoga still teaches in Mysore, Karnataka, India. His name is Sri K. Pattabhi Jois, but his students affectionately call him Guruji. In the winter of 1999–2000, I spent a little over two months in Mysore, studying with Guruji. It was as if I was spending time with the man who gave me a magic potion for happiness. At first I was blissed out just to be there. The very first day I met him, I awoke in the middle of the night and whispered, "I met Guruji." He is a jolly man, eighty-five years old, with bright eyes and a huge smile. I immediately felt an incredible amount of affection for him; this only continues to grow. His English is broken, but this seems to endear him even more to his students. Besides, his teaching is not derived from his words. Guruji often says, "Yoga is 99 percent practice, 1 percent theory." One can read text after text concerning yoga. One can write about yoga, talk about yoga, and think about yoga. But unless one does it, yoga is not happening. Guruji himself does not lecture about yoga. He teaches asanas and he makes jokes or talks about coffee. His knowledge of yoga philosophy is vast, but he insists that knowing is not understanding. The practice itself teaches us what we need.

"Do your practice, all is coming." These famous words of Sri K. Pattabhi Jois have traveled from Mysore to American magazines and hip yoga studios. This is a seemingly simple phrase, but *what* is coming? The asanas become easier. You might say they "come along." When I first started yoga, about four years ago, each pose was peculiar. Some poses were easy, others were very difficult. I would laugh and tumble or shake my head in awe at my teachers' graceful demonstrations. Then slowly, bit by bit, the primary series of Ashtanga yoga came. Yet there is always more to come: each asana can be perfected. I am working on the second series of asanas— and there are four more series! I know I will never reach the end, which is absolutely fine because perfection of asanas is not the goal.

Yoga is defined in Patanjali's *Yoga Sutras* as the cessation of the turnings of the mind. It is also a state of being in which one has transcended the material world and is absorbed in the soul or in God. At this point in my journey, I view yoga as a practice, a process that helps me to know myself so that I can move in the world with mindfulness, compassion, and friendliness. For theists such as myself, yoga is also a way to experience the sacred. I believe it all "comes" bit by bit. In the spirit of Guruji, I might say, "Slowly it is coming."

There are benefits to yoga. We tone our muscles, gain flexibility, cleanse organs. We do yoga for relaxation, stress release, peacefulness. All these are coming. Yet, I believe there is something beyond all that. Every day that I practice, revelations come: about myself, my relationships, answers to how I ought to conduct myself in this life. Often they are subtle. It may be a feeling or a slight lift in my mood. Sometimes I hardly even realize that something has shifted within me, but it has. I think it is about becoming attuned to the inner world, grounding oneself in the self or in God, then taking that centeredness into daily life and loving well. I have to keep practicing because it is so easy to move away from that space. However, not all that is coming is warm and fuzzy. Sometimes I realize how sad I am. Sometimes I don't even acknowledge my sadness intellectually, I just cry during or after practice. Yoga is about stopping thought. Yet stopping thought often involves facing all my thoughts and all my emotions. I cannot escape what is real in my present life. All is coming.

I can safely say I am happy with who I am and my life thus far. Yet I can also look at myself and see a jumbled mess of a human being. But when I practice yoga, whether I am with Guruji in Mysore, with my American teachers in California, or by myself amidst the clutter of my bedroom, I am sifting through myself. And things happen.

II.

On my first trip to India, I spent over an hour every afternoon for about four months with a yogi named Devadas Gandhi. Devadas lived in a little room on the grounds of the Gandhi Museum in Madurai, Tamil Nadu. He looked like the yogis I read about in books: he was thin to the point of emaciation, he wore only *kadhi* (homespun) cloth, his hair and beard had not been cut in years. His behavior was also what I would expect from a yogi— he talked slowly and carefully, and he always sat tall and often in *padmasana* (lotus posture, each ankle on the opposite thigh). His eyes communicated more than his words.

Each day we did about thirty or forty minutes of asanas. Devadas and I moved through postures on the roof of one of the buildings at the Gandhi Museum. We practiced on dirty old straw rugs under a thatched roof that supposedly helped block the southern Indian heat. We were surrounded by sounds of all sorts: auto rickshaws beeping, cows mooing, kids playing, women talking. There were often flies and mosquitoes disrupting my practice. The whole scene was vastly different from my yoga experiences in the United States. I often wondered how Devadas would react to our polished and temperature-controlled studios, our brightly colored sticky mats, and our expensive yoga outfits. My most basic lesson from Devadas was the confirmation that we don't need a studio and spandex in order to enjoy yoga.

Although the practice of asanas was not vigorous, it served its purpose: preparing me for meditation. After meditation, Devadas often read a page or two from a spiritual text—sometimes written by yogis or swamis, other times derived from a Quaker magazine or a Christian book. But even more profound than the readings was Devadas himself. Something special emanated from him; being in his presence was calming. Day after day, I sat there gazing at him, open and smiling, excitedly gobbling up anything he said, but also just feeling the internal alteration that occurred on these afternoons. He enjoyed slowly repeating phrases such as "Silence is the best conversation." He even had that phrase posted above his door. He also said things like, "Be your own light is the answer to every question." One day, I talked with him about my desire to go to the Sri Aurobindo Ashram in Pondicherry, where Devadas himself studied some years ago. I mentioned the reading I had been doing, I suppose trying to show him what I knew and to demonstrate my dedication. He answered, "Books are only information." He repeated himself slowly: "Books are only information." He continued, "Time is more important." Finally, he said, "A tree does not grow in a day."

As I reread these phrases in my journal several years later, I can't help but compare them to self-help books or envision them as bumper stickers right next to "Think Peace" on an old Volkswagen. But at the time, these words triggered an internal earthquake. That night my journal entry recorded my utter disorientation. Here I was, a college student studying in India. In addition to the reading I was doing for my classes, I had begun reading a number of yoga texts—some of which Devadas had given me. I was thinking, evaluating, criticizing, memorizing, ruminating, writing—I was approaching my study of yoga academically, the way I knew how. I was being a good American: I was actively *doing*! But "books are only information"? I suddenly began to realize the importance of experience, of letting things happen, of waiting for God. But this is not a story about an overachieving bookworm who leaves for an ashram (although I was deeply tempted by ashrams). I was never quite a pure academic, though I continue to study yoga texts. I still see the value in reading and intellectually engaging yoga philosophy. Nonetheless, something shifted for me that day. We can understand that it is important to be patient, that real life is more important than books, that the point of studying yoga is to understand it better to improve your own practice. But there is something very different about really knowing; heart-knowing as opposed to brain-knowing. Books don't have the answers: the soul does.

Being with Devadas was a journey to my soul. He taught me a lot with his words and his way of being, but it was mostly the feeling I had when practicing or sitting with him that affected me the most. I entered a space of calm; a calm that stayed with me on the streets of India. I can hardly describe what being calm all the time was like. I felt enveloped in peace and love. I enjoyed the external world but felt detached from it. My internal world was so huge, the external world diminished in importance. Readjusting to the United States was very difficult. In addition to amoebic dysentery, I struggled with the fast-paced American world. I went back to school, but for several months I didn't enjoy going out with friends. I remember wishing I could check out of my college life and check into an ashram somewhere. All I wanted was to do yoga, to meditate, and to be with God. School seemed ridiculous. But gradually that mind-set changed and I reclaimed my existence as a young college kid. I began going to parties again and by senior year I was obsessed with my thesis, which was on yoga. I embraced the external world of fun and books and wine and normal college activities. Then I graduated, and here I am, a year later, held in tension between the desire to be a normal twenty-two-year-old and the tendency toward the internal life. Underneath my worldly needs and wants, I know my soul thirsts for quiet—the kind of quiet I found on the roof of the Gandhi Museum, sweating, bitten by bugs, surrounded by beeps, moos, calls, and shouts.

Autumn Grace Jacobsen graduated from Vassar College in 1999 with a degree in religious studies. She has studied with and worked for the South India Term Abroad program in Tamil Nadu, India. On her second trip to India, Jacobsen studied Ashtanga yoga with Sri K. Pattabhi Jois. She practices yoga and finds jobs here and there, now and then. She currently lives in Santa Barbara, California.

It is like swallowing a red-hot iron ball.
You try to vomit it out, but you can't.

MUMONKAN

MERLE PENDELL

The Red-Hot Iron Ball

Last week, after returning from visiting a gravely ill friend, I was reflecting on what seems like a flood of recent deaths—my mother, my father, and four close friends. The late afternoon sunlight was shining on the altar I have in my dining room, and I remembered another late afternoon when the unthinkable, the unbearable, happened. Isaac, my beautiful, immortal firstborn son, had disappeared into 12 feet of fresh powder on the slopes of the Sierra Nevada, near Lake Tahoe. His body was found six hours later.

At that time I had been a practicing Buddhist for ten years. I really felt that I had "come home" when I was first introduced to Buddhism. I loved the teachings, the rituals, the calmness, and the Buddhist way of being in this life. I came to appreciate the different versions of the four vows that one learns from various teachers, or *roshis*. My favorite version remains the one Joko Beck uses:

> *Caught in the self-centered dream, only suffering;*
> *Holding to self-centered thoughts, exactly the dream;*
> *Each moment, life as it is, the only teacher;*
> *Being just this moment, compassion's way.*

I find myself saying at least one of these vows on many occasions. The vows and precepts, for me, are rich and powerful guides; so too, are some of the teaching stories I've heard in my practice.

One story in particular has become very important for me. In Mumonkan's *Comment on Case One, Chao-chou's Dog,* he says, "It is like swallowing a red-hot iron ball. You try to vomit it out, but you can't." With my son's death I found myself in that astonishing condition. No longer an abstract theory, it was as real as being struck by lightning. I had this red-hot iron ball in my mouth and I could not spit it out and I could not swallow it. I could not accept his death nor could I deny it. I remember feeling as if I was staggering around with this iron ball in my mouth and wondering how people could just walk by me. Couldn't they see?

It has taken several years for the raw grief to subside, for me to not feel so exposed, to be able to move in public without feeling the need to bolt home for safety. Bob Dylan's "Knockin' on Heaven's Door," sung at Isaac's memorial, can still bring me to my knees.

My altar has changed and grown over the years. It is now the repository, for the time being, of my son's ashes, my father's ashes, and small amounts of the ashes of dear friends. On *El Dia de Los Muertos* (Day of the Dead) the altar becomes a Mexican *ofrenda* filled with marigolds, pictures of dead friends and relatives, favorite foods and drinks, sugar skulls, and comical skeletons. It holds the first pomegranate and the first persimmon of the season as well as narcissus and daffodils, all favorites of my son. There were two green apples in Isaac's backpack the day he died, so throughout the year I will often place two green apples as an offering.

As I look at my altar now, seven years later, I have a deep and comforting realization. I have, indeed, swallowed that red-hot ball! It is lodged near my heart and it burns. It burns with a ferocity of love that is so intense I sometimes have to cry out, "Yes, yes, Isaac, I love you!"

Merle Pendell has studied Zen Buddhism with Aitken Roshi at Ring of Bone Zendo and at Ko-ko An; with Joko Beck at San Diego Zen Center; with Nelson Foster at Ring of Bone; at Santa Cruz Zen Center, and at Belly of the Beast Zendo. Like Jemimah Puddleduck, she is "not a very good sitter" but she perseveres. Pendell lives in Santa Cruz, California.

The Mind is always busy criticizing and arguing;
rather, the basis of your actions should be love.

IQBAL, PAKISTANI POET-PHILOSOPHER

※

WAHEED SIDDIQEE

The Wisdom of Mothers, Poets, and Saints

WHEN I WAS A CHILD, I ALWAYS ASKED MY MOTHER TO TELL ME A STORY BEFORE going to sleep. She would tell me a little anecdote, a short story, or a proverb. Later in life, I realized that many of her wise and compassionate sayings have woven a continuous thread of inspiration all through my life.

One of my favorite stories is about a widow who owned a little vegetable shop and her young daughter who helped her run it. The daughter had a sincere lover. One day the mother told her daughter to attend to customers while she cleaned the back of the shop. Shortly thereafter the daughter's lover happened to stop by and wanted to purchase some vegetables. The daughter, finding herself in the presence of her lover, was so overwhelmed that she kept putting vegetables in her lover's basket without counting or weighing them. When the mother noticed what her daughter was doing, she called her and said, "Oh my dear daughter, are you keeping any account of how much you are giving away?" To this the daughter replied, "Oh Mother, what account? Who keeps account of the beloved?" At that very moment a pious person was passing by, reciting the name of God using a string of beads to help him count. As he heard what the daughter said, he threw away the beads and shouted in ecstasy "What great thought! What deep insight! She knows the true meaning of love! Here I am counting how many times I have recited the name of God! What narrow insight I have about love compared to this young girl."

Other sources of my inspiration about love and wisdom include the lives and writings of the mystic saints Rabia Basri and Jalaluddin Rumi, a Sufi[1] mystic, as well as those of the poet philosopher Iqbal.

Once someone asked Rabia Basri whether she hated Satan. She replied, "No, the love of God and His creation has left no room for the hatred of Satan." She would often urge, "I do not serve God for any reward—have no fear of hell or love of paradise. I am duty bound to serve Him only for His love."

Here are two of my favorite stories from the writings of Rumi.

The Man and the Bear

One day while a man was passing through a forest, he saw a serpent rushing to attack a bear. The man went to the aid of the bear, killed the serpent, and saved the bear. The bear was much moved by the kindness of the man. It followed him wherever he went and became his faithful slave. One day the man lay to rest under a shady tree. Soon he was asleep. The bear sat by his side to keep watch. Some flies came and sat on the face of the man. The bear drove them away. The flies came again and the bear drove them away again. The flies became so persistent that in his annoyance the bear lost patience. He took a large stone and hurled it at the flies, hoping to kill them. The flies, of course, escaped but the stone crushed the man to death. The moral of the story is, "Do not make friends with fools," for foolish friends may be more dangerous than your enemy.

The Mouse and the Camel

Once a mouse came across a nose string to which a camel was tied. The mouse got hold of the string, and as it moved, the camel moved with it. The mouse felt that it had become strong enough to move a camel. The mouse moved on and the camel followed it. The mouse felt proud that it had become so strong that even an animal such as a camel was obliged to follow it. The mouse spoke commanding words to the camel, but the camel kept quiet. It was thinking about teaching a lesson to the mouse. After they had traveled for some distance, a river came their way. Now the mouse hesitated to move forward. The camel wanted it to proceed, but the mouse said that if it proceeded it was likely to drown. The camel said that the water was not deep, and it could easily cross. The mouse said that the water might not be deep for the camel, but it was for the mouse. The camel then said, "If that is the case, why did you become so arrogant on coming to hold my nose string?" The mouse now realized its mistake. It apologized to the camel, and promised to behave humbly in the future.

This simple story always reminds me that one should never become arrogant, particularly if one happens to have a temporary advantage over others.

The poet-philosopher Iqbal has written many inspiring poems and essays pertaining to love and wisdom. Much of his writing is in Urdu, the national language of Pakistan. Some of his sayings that have had a deep influence on me include: "The mind is always busy criticizing and arguing; rather, the basis of your actions should be love." "True political life begins, not with demanding your rights, but with fulfilling your responsibilities." "Success in life depends on resolve—not on intelligence." "Life has innumerable stages. Many aspects of life are beyond human intellect. The insight and the understanding about such aspects comes through some other means. These means are not related to philosophy."

From my mother and from these poets and saints, I have learned that one goes through life constantly learning new lessons. There is so much we do not know.

---

[1] Sufism, a Muslim philosophical and literary movement, emerged in the late tenth and early eleventh centuries, borrowing ideas from Neoplatonism, Buddhism, and Christianity.

Originally from Pakistan, **Waheed Siddiqee, Ph.D.** became a United States citizen in 1973. He is chairman of the Interfaith Committee, United Muslims of America (a sociopolitical organization). He works with many interfaith groups on such issues as economic and social justice. Dr. Siddiqee was instrumental in arranging courses on Islam at the Graduate Theological Union in Berkeley, California. He is married with two sons and five grandchildren.

The practitioner who focuses on mindfulness
Advances like a fire,
Consuming the chains of bondage
Both great and small.

THE BUDDHA

SOGYAL RINPOCHE

Mindfulness in Everyday Life

THERE IS A STORY THAT I REMEMBER HEARING IN MY CHILDHOOD IN TIBET, ABOUT an old woman who came to the Buddha and asked him how to meditate. He told her to remain mindful, present, and aware of every movement of her hands as she drew the water from the well each day, knowing that if she did so, she would soon find herself in that state of alert and spacious calm that is meditation. The practice of mindfulness, simple yet powerful, is the heart of meditation, and the supreme antidote to distraction. For, as the Buddha taught, the root of all our suffering is ignorance, but the root of ignorance itself is our mind's habitual tendency to distraction. So mindfulness is the gateway to liberation. Buddha said:

> *The practitioner who focuses on mindfulness*
> *Advances like a fire,*
> *Consuming the chains of bondage*
> *Both great and small.*

What is it then that mindfulness brings? It allows all the warring and fragmented aspects of ourselves to settle and become friends; it gradually defuses our negativity; and it removes the unkindness in us, revealing our true nature, our compassionate Good Heart. One of my masters, Nyoshul Khen Rinpoche, calls mindfulness "the fortress of the mind" and "the friend of wisdom," for in its magical simplicity come a presence and a peace which are sane and grounded, clear, joyful, and awake, and full of compassion and wisdom.

When I first began to teach in the West, I found to my surprise that many spiritual practitioners today lack the knowledge of how to integrate their meditation practice with everyday life. But nothing could be more important. It cannot be said too strongly or too often: to integrate meditation in action is the whole ground and point and purpose of meditation. Here, too, mindfulness holds the key, for the true discipline of meditation is to maintain the thread of mindfulness throughout our everyday life. It is the continual application of that presence of mind that can bring about a deep change in a person's life and become a source of real healing. Isn't it extraordinary, though, how difficult it is, as we go about our lives, simply to remember to be mindful and to bring the mind home whenever we catch ourselves lost in distraction? I created a slogan, which my students find helpful: *Remember to remember, when you remember.*

So to integrate meditation with life, the Buddhist masters tell us there is no substitute for regular practice, for only through real practice will we be able to taste unbrokenly the calm of our true nature of mind, and so be able to sustain the experience of it in our everyday life. That is why developing stability in spiritual practice is so important, through first practicing in the right environment and in proper practice sessions and then mixing the experience of practice with everyday life.

Sogyal Rinpoche was born in Tibet and raised by one of the most esteemed spiritual masters of this century, Jamyang Khyentse Chokyi Lodro. He travels and lectures throughout the world and is the founder and spiritual director of Rigpa, a network of Buddhist centers and groups.

You have your own experiences, your own unique perspective
that no one else can give to this work.
You write it from there, you work from there,
and when or where it manifests, that is His concern.

SRIPADA BABA

E. H. RICK JAROW

Sripada

"WE'VE GOT TO GET GANESH, YOU NEED THIS GANESH TO HELP YOU FINISH YOUR dissertation." Sripada (pronounced "shree-pad") said it, and that generally was it. Devotees, like pawns on a chessboard, would move into action: someone would go to the phone, someone would make tea, and someone else would bring in a car. Not just servants, but high government officials would come, with their own servants, to meet with this wild-looking man-creature who wore nothing but a thin, soiled yellow cloth wrapped around his body like an Indian toga. Sripada never wore shoes, coats, rings, or watches, and there was not a shred of adornment on his body, unless you counted his matted hair, dreadlocks almost down to his waist in *sadhu* fashion.

A *sadhu,* indeed, he was. Sripada Baba was one of the most charismatic and enigmatic holy men to appear in the north Indian area, known as Braj, in years. At his funeral some people would say that they did not know if he was a saint or a demon, for there were all sorts of stories about him, good, bad, and ugly; and who knew what to believe? But there was one type of story that was consistently told by almost everyone who had any sustained contact with him: if you had a plan, Sripada would disrupt it; if you had an idea of how things were going to be, Sripada would change it; if you were trying to hide anything (your self included), Sripada would find it; and if you were holding on to something, Sripada would take it.

43

There was one story about a *mahatma*, a holy seer living in a mountain cave, writing poems to the divine. The *mahatma* ate next to nothing, lived on scraps of food that visitors and nature provided, and had no possessions save his poems. Sripada Baba came to see him, stayed with him for awhile in blissful communion, and then took off with the poems. The *mahatma*, agitated and distraught, came down from his mountain searching for Sripada and the poems, but never found either of them.

Braj is the short name for the area around the holy city of Brindaban, the place where the Divine eternally manifests in the forms of Radha and Krishna, the divine lovers whose grace overflows throughout creation. "Sripada" literally means "at the feet of Sri." *Sri*, in this case, indicates the Goddess Radha, whose selfless love is the key to *bhakti*, the highest form of spiritual ecstasy. To be at the feet of Sri, is to ever be at the wellspring of *ananda cinmaya rasa vigraha*, the flowing form of inspired bliss. But Sripada, more often than not, displayed his divine opulences in curious ways.

I remember when I was in Brindaban on an academic grant and may have had the only computer in town. Sripada found me, of course, and soon had me typing letter after letter to government officials protesting the air and water pollution of various holy places along the Ganges and demanding action.

The electricity could go out in Brindaban at any time. This was not uncommon in small towns in India, and like the heat and dust, it was something you learned to live with. And repeatedly, just when it seemed that I would finally finish one of the letters, the current would shut down and my letter would evaporate along with other materials on my disk. Now, I had done some work with South American shamans back in the States who saw things like this in terms of spirits. So I mentioned to Sripada that perhaps there were some negative spirits in the area who were blocking the completion of the work. "The only negative spirit here," said Sripada, looking at me sternly, "is if I am not sincere."

We worked on through the night. One of the things Sripada was celebrated for was that he did not seem to require sleep. He would remain up for weeks, twenty-four hours a day, unfazed by any physical needs. Then he would hibernate somewhere for awhile and return. I once actually saw him sleeping on a roof (in northern India the summers are so hot that everyone sleeps up on a roof to avoid baking). I was on a high roof, and I saw Sripada on a lower one. It was about four in the morning. In my whole life to this day, I have never seen anyone asleep like that. It was as if "no one was home." He did not move a muscle, not a twitch, hardly even a breath. There was total serenity, utter calm and stillness. I sensed for a moment what the Upanishads meant when they spoke of the "dreamless sleep" as a merging back into the infinite Brahman.

Sripada kept me up typing all night. I was cursing him under my breath as everyone did when he got you, and that seemed to be his game plan. He would find you, ask you to do some seemingly innocent task, and then he would get you. He would get you anxious, disturbed, and ultimately out of control, as he held a mirror up to your clinging ego.

There were all sorts of stories about him: his yelling, his beating, his roaming the countryside. He had once told an aspiring yogi to come take a short walk with him and to bring a toothbrush. He brought the yogi back three months later. Another time, he remained waist-deep in the freezing Ganges on a pilgrimage expedition, transfixed in meditation for eight hours, while everyone else had no choice but to wait.

At five in the morning, as the temple bells were ringing, the letters were finally finished. As he got ready to leave and I was thinking, "Thank goodness he's finally gone and I can now get some sleep," he turned to me with a queer smile over his one chipped tooth and said softly, "Congratulations, you have won a small victory over *tamas*." *Tamas* means "dark inertia" in Sanskrit and is associated with indolence, lethargy, and sleep. I found that I did not need to sleep at all that day, and I couldn't help but wonder if he had staged this entire scenario to show me that I really did not need the sleep I thought I did, to demonstrate what was possible.

So when Sripada told me we were going to get a Ganesh (meaning a statue of the elephant god, Ganesha, the lord of thresholds and remover of obstacles) to help me finish my dissertation, I couldn't help wondering what the punch line was going to be. He didn't have to sucker you in; he drew you in with his charismatic power until it was too late and you realized that you were in for one of his rides to God knows where.

Sripada, it is said, had been a boy saint. When he was fifteen years old and riding on a bus, he would have to put a blanket over his head at every stop because if the people saw him they would run after him. He had left home at the age of eight because he realized that the teachers in his school would never be able to teach him how to control his mind. So he walked out of his birth home and began to wander. He met a *rishi* who had him tending cows in a pasture for a number of years. He had meditated up in the mountains and had all the trappings of a renunciate. But somewhere along the line something had happened—he had been bitten by *radha-bhava,* the mood of devotion and absolute love that the goddess Radha has for the god Krishna. And he had come to Brindaban, the home of love and devotion, the town where Krishna had spent his youth, where the very dust is said to be made of pure love. And there he had exhibited all the symptoms of *mahabhava,* the fullness of divine joy. So much so, that when he was residing in an ashram, they always had someone keep watch over him. He would be cooking for Radha, would go into a trance, and leave his hand in the fire.

Everyone in the town respected him, revered him, or was afraid of him. He hardly looked human, with his matted hair and chipped teeth, walking slowly without a care in the outer world. The angle on the Ganesh turned out to be this: He decided that we had to go to Delhi to get a very particular silver Ganesh icon that was made by a particular silversmith somewhere in the bowels of *chandi-chowk,* the old silver market. To go there we were going to borrow the white Toyota of my colleagues, the Jamesons, who were employed in the United States embassy in Delhi. A Toyota in Delhi at that time was like a Rolls Royce, but these Americans were liberal, open minded, and even inquisitive. They were drawn in by the myths of the holy men; and moreover they trusted me, a Fulbright scholar from Columbia University. "Sure," they said. "He can have the Toyota and the driver, but please bring it back by six in the evening because we have an important government function to attend."

And Baba said, "Of course," and had tea with them and vibed them and off we went. We circled around Delhi for hours, going from one little market to another. Baba never bothered with such trivialities as time, but as it got closer and closer to six, I started squirming, giving off little hints, and finally said to Baba that we *had* to bring the car back at six. No answer. Six o'clock came and went. It was now 7:30. Baba didn't speak, he just kept directing the driver to one site after another. I was beside myself, looking for a phone or any way to get them a message, feeling guilty and angry at his callousness and lack of respect for anything and anyone. It was eight o'clock when we found the Ganesh he wanted, nine by the time we got it. Naturally the craftsman offered it to Baba with great fanfare and devotion, which included a half-hour tea session. It was 9:45 when we returned to the Jamesons. No one was home. I couldn't sit still, I was so filled with anxiety. By the time the Jamesons returned at 10:30, I was beside myself, just waiting for the storm, the tirade. But there was nothing. It turned out that they had not needed the Toyota that evening and everything had arranged itself perfectly. Baba just looked at me, no words, and disappeared into the shadows. I would not see him again for three years.

Some twelve years after that incident, I was typing up the last chapter of a book that had come from the dissertation research done in India at that time. The Ganesh was on my bookcase behind my desk. I was way past my deadline and was harried and hurried and beside myself. Would they accept the book as it was? Should I ask for an extension? I looked at the Ganesh and suddenly it struck me. Maybe Baba had orchestrated this as well to teach me something; that time was fluid, that expectations are conditional, and that what had to be done would and could be done in its own time. I remembered how at one point I was so discouraged with my work that I was going to quit. Sripada appeared in my compound that evening and asked what I was up to. I told him that I was quitting my dissertation work because I've run into eight-year-olds who know more Sanskrit than me. I'm slogging through my dictionaries and I see kids citing entire volumes by heart. "That may be true," he said, "but that is not what is important. You have your own experiences, your own unique perspective that no one else can give to this work. You write it from there, you work from there, and when or where it manifests, that is His concern." He made a gesture in the air that it was God's concern. You do the work, you work with your heart, you work so attentively that time stops. And suddenly you are no longer working against the clock or against someone's deadline. You are in the *bhav*, you are in the mood of it; and then it can happen. Then Ganesh, the remover of obstacles, appears, in the bowels of a dirty, grimy city, in the center of your confusion. Everything aligns from that center, not from how you thought it was or should be, but how it all is. I said thank you twelve years later.

E. H. Rick Jarow is assistant professor of history of religions at Vassar College, former Mellon Fellow in the Humanities at Columbia University, resident of Braj academy in Vrindaban, India, practicing career consultant, and teacher of meditation. Jarow is the author of *Creating the Work You Love: Courage, Commitment, and Career, In Search of the Sacred, Your Life's Work, Opening to Shakti,* and numerous articles and talks. His seminars on "career and soul" focus on interfacing intuitive experience with effective action.

At every stage of my journey, the beautiful word *ehipassiko*
became my song, my direction.
Whatever was happening, I heard myself called
to come and see for myself:
Is *this* true?

WENDY EGYOKU NAKAO

Come and See

EHIPASSIKO. COME AND SEE. THIS IS AN ANCIENT WORD THAT COMES FROM PALI, a language that lives today in the melodic chants of Buddhists. *Ehipassiko* has been a life-turning word for me. I heard it chanted for the very first time while on a three-month meditation retreat. Sitting deep in the autumn-colored maple woods of New England, the melody of this invitation pierced my heart. A door opened. I heard the Buddha's voice inviting me: "Come. Come here. Come to now." At this gentle beckoning, I stepped into my life.

It is not possible to ever step outside of one's life. But at that time, I didn't know this, for I felt quite apart from everything, inadequate and unfulfilled. Something was missing. I had embarked on a journey to find the missing pieces of myself. At every stage of my journey, the beautiful word *ehipassiko* became my song, my direction. Whatever was happening, I heard myself called to come and see for myself: Is *this* true? "Look," the song said, "right here, now. Plunge into life as it is. Life is coming into being. Life is leaving. Take care, take care."

I recall one day in particular when this invitation pierced my veil of self-preoccupation. While in her early sixties, my mother showed the first signs of what became a long illness, during which she lost her ability to speak and move. As far as we could tell, her mind was intact. My father and younger brother became her devoted caregivers. During one of my visits home, I saw the difficulties my family members were enduring in the day-to-day care of our mother. At the same time, I marveled at their meticulous caretaking of her. Here, again, was the invitation. Without complaint, my father had plunged into what was for him the bewildering and foreign worlds of the household and round-the-clock care of a sick person—preparing meals, cleaning and more cleaning, changing our mother's diapers, feeding her, lifting and turning the leaden weight of his bedridden wife.

One day, my father, taking advantage of the respite my presence gave him, went out to play the Japanese card game *sakura* with his friends. In the morning, we had sat my mother in a chair. As evening approached and he had not yet returned, I became increasingly aware of the length of time she had been sitting and of the necessity of moving her. I was not sure I could move her by myself. As I grew more and more anxious, I found myself caught in a maelstrom of fear and self-doubt: Where is he? How long can we keep taking care of her like this? What are we going to do? Is she ever going to die?

In the midst of this mental anguish, I explained to my mother that I was going to move her. With all my might, I picked her up, struggling to keep her upright, and slowly inched her toward the bed. She leaned heavily on me in complete abandon and trust. Miraculously, we reached the bed and, in a heap, fell onto it together. I could not really tell from her eyes what she might have been thinking, but then I heard my own laughter. "Mom," I laughed, "*Everything* is as it is. Even *this!*"

The Buddha's invitation always brings me back to now, to *this* moment—whatever is happening. *Ehipassiko* demands of me, "Now that you are here, what will you do?" My life is intimate with the trees, the animals, the earth, the sky, all beings. But "with" is not enough. This is a no-gap intimacy. My life *is* tree, flower, sunset, garbage, stars, and moon, all suffering human beings—the crying child, the crippled old person, the anxious new mother, the distressed, the sick, the poor, the ones who hurt others, the incapacitated loved one. The no-gap intimacy insists that I respond by coming into this truth and seeing what needs to be done. How can I serve this life that I *am?*

Ehipassiko is an invitation for me to investigate the joys and sufferings of life, but it is not merely a technique that I remember and employ. *Ehipassiko* is constantly turning me, readjusting and repositioning me, so that I cannot ignore this life that I *am.* My very being turns on my active acceptance of what is and my capacity to love another. Sometimes it is a struggle: I do not wish to be turned. I want to ignore the suffering, just as I did not wish to witness my mother withering into a shadow. At those times, I feel myself shrinking into a small and self-centered person, content with fulfilling my own needs. But then, again, the veil is raised—sometimes by a cold wind, a homeless person asking for a quarter, or the persistent cries of a mockingbird. I am beckoned to the present: "*Come.* Come outside of your narrow self-enclosure and step into life."

When I first heard the beautiful word *ehipassiko,* I found a gem of love and clarity among the colored leaves of a crisp New England autumn. It reflects the myriad forms of life, appearing now ruby red, at other times the green jade of growth, the brown of decay, or the all-encompassing blue of sky. This gem continuously illuminates all my missing pieces.

Now, *you* come and see for yourself. Is *this* true?

Wendy Egyoku Nakao began practicing *zazen* in 1975, when a friend dared her to plunge into a seven-day *sesshin* (Zen retreat). She was ordained as a Theravadan nun by Tungpalu Sayadaw in Bodhi Gaya, India, and later in the Zen tradition by Taizan Maezumi Roshi, founding abbot of the Zen Center of Los Angeles. She is a Dharma successor of Roshi Bernie Glassman and is presently abbot and head teacher of the Zen Center of Los Angeles.

"Funny child, you want so badly to know such things, yet it is clear that you don't even know where you stand now," said the master. "That's silly, master, I am standing here with you, by these trees." "And where is that, exactly?" retorted the master.

FROM A TAOIST PARABLE

JOHN ADAMS

Lost in Movement, Found in Stillness

WE'RE ALL LOST IN SPACE, AND NO MATTER HOW MUCH WE MEDITATE WE WILL never be able to fully comprehend where exactly we are and why. It is this hopeless, optimistic viewpoint that allows me to relax and enjoy the ride. Taoist meditation (Tao: the way, the path) and *qigong* (internal energy work) serve to both humor and humble the aspects of my being that feel a compulsion to know precise truth. Taoism helps me feel more connected and compassionate and it reminds me that I am just another player in life who belongs to nature and the natural order. After all, the secrets of the Tao are unknowable. Some truths and secrets can be discovered, but some cannot. I think a certain part of our nature understands deeper truths, but our everyday consciousness has been programmed to ignore these layers of reality, including the seemingly unknowable reality of our existence. The only thing I feel certain about is that during meditation, I often feel the sense of being in many places simultaneously, and that my normal, localized consciousness gets replaced by something else.

So far, one of the most liberating gifts of my practice has been the "I don't know much of anything" epiphanies I get whenever I choose to look and listen with a calm mind and still body. The more I practice my Taoist meditation, the more lost in space I feel. Part of me rejoices and is delighted by the adventure, mystery, and awesome powers that flow through and around me as I practice. However, sometimes a glimpse into the unknown sets my ego and mind into a tailspin of confusion, doubt, insecurity, and self-pity.

There is a particular story told to me by my Baguazhang (eight-diagram palm-boxing art) teacher, Dr. John Painter, Sifu (head teacher) Daoqiquan (way of internal boxing), that has had that dual effect on me for many years now. The impatient beginner student wanted to know the secret of cultivating internal power and asked his Taoist master for more advanced material. The master laughed at him and said, "You are practicing the advanced material now but you're new at it and therefore blind to its truth and essence."

The student insisted once more that he was ready to understand more advanced spiritual concepts. Again the master laughed at him and with a kindly yet mischievous grin initiated the student into oblivion with the following dialogue:

"Funny child, you want so badly to know such things, yet it is clear that you don't even know where you stand now," said the master.

"That's silly, master, I am standing here with you, by these trees."

"And where is that, exactly?" retorted the master.

"In your backyard, in Texas. Hey, I know where we are, okay!" replied the frustrated student.

"Where's that?" asked the master again.

"In the southern United States."

"Where's that?" responded the master casually.

"On the North American continent! What's the point of this?"

"Where's the North American continent?" asked the master harshly.

The student paused a moment and tried to regain his composure so as to not lash out verbally at the crazy old master.

"North America is on Earth," he replied in deep frustration.

"Where's that?"

"Third planet from the sun, Milky Way galaxy," said the student triumphantly. The master gave the young student no slack.

"Great, and where exactly is that?"

The young man finally got the picture and admitted defeat.

"I don't know where it is, master."

"Exactly. See, you are truly lost. You have no idea where you are and yet you insist on having me show you the secrets of the Tao. Go finish your standing practice for today, repeat daily for one hundred days in a row, and come back to see me when you have completed this task. Then you might know better where you stand and be ready to accept the play of Daoqiquan!"

The best solution for my serious-minded, restless ego is to remember that all practice must be *played*. In fact, all life must be played. A big part of what attracted me to Chinese martial and health arts is that practitioners refer to themselves as players, not fighters. I had had enough of fighting and wanted to play and rejoice in life. I have found that when playing a particular action or circumstance, I enjoy all the various actions and businesses of living. This is not a casual or flip approach, but rather a more reverent and challenging one. Since I am perpetually lost, I might as well relax and enjoy the ride that life provides, toward a destination of joy, gratitude, and humility.

When I play Jiulong Baguazhang, my ego tends to melt into the void and is replaced by a different version of me. In both circle walking and standing still, the specific *Yijing gua* element images that I create in my mind take over and seem to play with my body. The specific images for Heaven, Earth, Lake, and Wind each have a life of their own somewhere inside my consciousness. I am their host, not their master. I let them into my house and offer the fruits of my mental and physical play, and they show me how to furnish and decorate it and help me add new rooms.

I don't know where they come from, these energies specific to each *gua* image, but I do know they are inside me from time to time when I call on them. To them I am not lost, not hurtling endlessly though space. These eternal energies find life inside and around my consciousness. They exist like multidimensional movies inside my imagination at first and later become part of my physical structure as well. My nervous system learns to associate specific images and feelings to the prescribed movements of each *gua*. This creates unique energetic qualities for each *gua* movement I perform. Yet, I don't really do them. They do me. They come out and play like wise old rascal dragons, lovingly and powerfully coiling, wrapping, soaring, swimming, gracefully creating and destroying each new moment.

It is in this play that I happily lose myself for awhile and remember that I can experience so much more of life's gifts when I let go of the need to know and the need to control. I am just as lost as I was years ago, but today I fully accept this fact and am open to catching more glimpses of infinity. Most days I feel less need to take myself so seriously. This is one of the greatest gifts that these Taoist practices have afforded me.

Being accountable for how I perceive and how I respond seems easier as a result of my practice. Maybe it's serenity or peace of mind, or maybe it's just growing up and having greater acceptance and reverence. Whatever it is, it's not where I am or why that matters anymore, it's how I create and play each moment. I have more fun these days and I strongly believe this is due in large part to my play with those powerful Baguazhang dragons.

John Adams is a long-time practitioner of both internal and external martial arts. He is a Silver Glove instructor of Boxe Française Savate and is California's Jiulong Baguazhang Heaven Palm instructor under Dr. John Painter (Sifu Daoqiquan). Adams works professionally as a certified Neurostructural Integration Technique therapist and is the founder and director of the Internal Arts Center in Santa Monica, California.

Form is emptiness, emptiness is form,
everything that is form is emptiness,
everything that is emptiness form.

There are no eyes no ears no nose no tongue no body and no mind.
There is no color no sound no smell no taste no touch no mental object.

There is nothing to have and the mind is no hindrance.
Gone, gone, gone, completely gone, gone beyond everything.

FROM THE *HEART SUTRA*

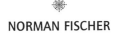

NORMAN FISCHER

My Mother

AT FIRST IT WAS A SHOCK TO SEE HER. SHE DIDN'T LOOK THE SAME AT ALL. HER face was ashen and all puffed up from the chemotherapy and radiation, her arms were huge from it, her hair was matted, scarce, and a different color, her voice had gone all croaky and harsh, and the medication had got her mixed up and disconnected. She'd sit up in bed all of a sudden, beside herself with anger or frustration, and yell to my Aunt Adeline, "No, turn me over, not that way this way, no not that way I said like this, like that," and my poor Aunt Adeline would try to be helpful but nothing was helpful. Adeline and my father and my Aunt Sylvia all looked at one another and me. Their look expressed an unspecified and very confused dismay.

She'd go in and out of consciousness. She'd see things. She said, "Don't let them make you do anything you don't want to."

She said, "You all think I'm crazy but I know what I'm doing."

She said, "Throw away all the envelopes that you can."

She said, "Why are you all standing around here? It's ridiculous! Scram!"

And she said to me, "You're a cute boy in that shirt."

After a while it was very beautiful to see her so earnestly living this simple, intense, painful, but somehow noble existence in the 6-foot-by-3-foot space of hospital bed that was her whole life. There and the unknown realms of space and time through which she traveled.

She said, "Put my shoes in boxes over there."

We'd take shifts staying with her around the clock, and I would look forward very much to being with her, to be able to be as intimate with her as I had been as a child and to have a clearer and purer relationship to her than I had been able to have for many, many years. She had been for a long time disappointed in my life. She loved me very much and I think felt frustrated in something in her life and so needed me to afford her satisfaction in some way. But I never did that. I had an unusual kind of life. It was very hard for her. But now I could stroke her forehead and try to release the tension I could see building up around her eyes. And I could breathe with her and my doing that would calm her down a little bit. Sometimes, if she were making noise in her breathing, I'd make noise in the same way. But I couldn't do that when the others were around because it would make them nervous, as though I were doing some kind of voodoo. Sometimes she'd sit up suddenly out of her unconsciousness and say to me, "Don't make fun of me." And I'd say, "I'm not making fun of you. I love you." And late at night I could look at her in the lamplight and could think of how many ways I could have been nicer to her, and how much she'd loved me and given to me, and I could tell her how much I loved her and it would make me cry gently. And when she'd suddenly sit up and say, "My hat," or, "Get my shoes, we're going out," or "Where are the red and green charts? They should be up by now," I'd tell her, "Don't worry about that. Your life is very simple now. Just breathe." And she'd lie back down and feel calmer and reassured.

Gradually during the days and nights she began to give everything up. First, her body became more relaxed, as though it weren't hers anymore. Then, she stopped having any sense of whether she liked or didn't like anything. Then, she couldn't tell who anyone was or what anything was in the room. Then, all the worries and cares of her life began swimming around in her delirium, her clothes, things she had to do at home or for my father, things at the office where she worked, and one by one she put them down too. Finally there was only a dim awareness that got finer and finer as her breath seemed to go more and more deep, more and more inward. The heavy earth of her body dissolved into water. The water of the moving of her blood dissolved into the first of the images that receded in the distance. The fiery images dissolved into air and the air into space, endless space and endless consciousness.

My father cried and said, "It isn't fair," as my sons, arguing with one another or carefully watching each other divide some special food, often say. It isn't fair.

I knew she was gone, but it didn't really make sense that she was gone. Because she didn't go anywhere. And the gone that she was was really no different from the gone that she had usually been to me my whole adult life and even, a little bit more and more each day, in my life as a child. In one way she was gone. But in another she was very present. We stood there looking at her. She looked very noble and we were all in awe of her. Then everyone wanted to leave and I said, "Is it all right if I stay with her awhile?" and everyone said yes it was all right and they left.

It was nearly dawn. The light coming in the window was lovely and my mother looked lovely in the light. Her skin was a different color than it had been before. It looked very, very soft and gentle. I could see that she had many freckles on her face. I had never noticed before that she had freckles. I felt like talking to her. I said, "Don't be confused!"

Then I quietly recited the Heart Sutra. It says, "Form is emptiness, emptiness is form, everything that is form is emptiness, everything that is emptiness form." And it says, "There are no eyes no ears no nose no tongue no body and no mind. There is no color no sound no smell no taste no touch no mental object." And it says, "There is nothing to have and the mind is no hindrance." And it ends, "Gone, gone, gone, completely gone, gone beyond everything." I have recited this sutra thousands of times but I never felt so clearly as now what it meant.

I looked out the window. The Florida hospital lawns were pale green in the dawn light, very quiet and pure, as if brand new, with no one around. My mother was all right. She had everything she needed. Far away on the lawn a workman appeared and tried to start a lawn mower. It took many pulls before he got it going. And then silently and slowly he began pushing it back and forth across the lawn. Mama was all right. But it was going to be hard for the world with all its struggle and fragility and beauty to get along without her, and then I cried a lot for the world that didn't know any peace and perhaps never would.

Norman Fischer is a poet and Zen Buddhist priest. He served as co-abbot of the San Francisco Zen Center from 1995 to 2000. He is presently a senior Dharma teacher there as well as the founder and spiritual director of the Everyday Zen Foundation. Fischer has published several books of poetry, including *The Narrow Roads of Japan* (1998) and *Success* (2001). He is also the author of a prose memoir, *Jerusalem Moonlight* (1995), and *Racism: What About It?* which he coauthored with a group of African-American high school students. He lives with his wife, Kathie, in Muir Beach, California.

By virtue of this generosity may I achieve the great enlightenment
for the benefit of all kind mother sentient beings.

FROM A TIBETAN BUDDHIST PARABLE

GESHE TSULTIM GYELTSEN

The Buddha's Great Heart

THE DHARMA IS A METHOD OF TRANSFORMING OUR MINDS AND HEARTS. YOU and I wish only for happiness and do not want pain and suffering. When we know what causes happiness and what causes misery, only then can we begin the transformation of our body, speech, and mind. As it is stated in a *sutra:*

> *Abandon negativity;*
> *Practice virtue well;*
> *Subdue your mind:*
> *This is the Buddha's teaching.*

A Buddha's compassion is completely unbiased and without discrimination. For eons the Buddha accumulated merit through the practice of loving-kindness and compassion. There are countless stories that illustrate the magnificence of the Buddhas and Bodhisattvas. I would like to share two of them with you that were favorites in my family.

Buddha's Cousin

Devadatta was the jealous cousin of Shakyamuni Buddha. He always criticized and challenged the Buddha, never recognizing Buddha's positive actions. There was a great physician who offered an extremely potent nutritional pill to the Buddha. Devadatta knew of this and asked the doctor, "Why do you offer such medicine to the Buddha and not to me?" The doctor replied, "Such medicine is unsuitable for you." Devadatta answered, "There is no difference between the Buddha and me." After continuous requests, the doctor consented but offered only a quarter of the amount that he offered the Buddha. Devadatta insisted, however, that he receive the same amount. The doctor told Devadatta, "Such an amount would be too powerful; you will surely overdose and die. The Buddha and you are not equal!" Devadatta became annoyed; he believed there was not any difference between his knowledge and the Buddha's. He demanded the full amount, and so the doctor hesitantly gave it to him. As Devadatta swallowed the pill, he dropped to the ground and was on the brink of death. The omniscient Buddha directly perceived what was happening and appeared at his cousin's side. The Buddha placed his hand on Devadatta's head and said, "My dear cousin always criticizes me. However, my love for my son Rahula and my love for Devadatta are equal. If this statement is true, may Devadatta be healed." The Buddha gave the Power of Truth and immediately Devadatta was restored to perfect health.

As Devadatta regained consciousness, he saw the Buddha's hand on his head and rudely responded, "Why, Gautama [Buddha], is your hand on my head? Take it off!"

Three Princes

Once upon a time, there was a king and a queen who had three sons. The three princes were named Great God, Great Sound, and Great Heart. They had a day off from their studies and decided to take a field trip to the forest. As they reached their destination, they saw a mother tiger with her five cubs that looked frail and weak and were about to die. The brother Great Sound asked, "What type of food do they eat?" The older brother answered, "The tiger and her cubs live on the flesh and blood of others." The brother Great Sound replied, "This is an opportunity to practice generosity by giving the body. But I am incapable of doing this." The younger brother Great Heart felt deep sympathy and he thought to himself, "Numberless lives have passed without any meaning or essence; this time life shall not be wasted. I will offer my body as an act of generosity to the mother tiger and her five cubs." As Great Heart had such thoughts the earth trembled and the sky dulled as the sun eclipsed. The older brother became frightened and urged the others to return to the palace at once.

The older brother, Great God, led the way. Following behind him were Great Sound and the younger brother Great Heart. After a while, Great Heart stopped and returned to the mother tiger and her cubs. Great Heart removed his clothes, lay down in front of the mother tiger and her cubs, and prayed, "By virtue of this generosity may I achieve the great enlightenment for the benefit of all kind mother sentient beings." Moved by Great Heart's overwhelming compassion, the mother tiger and her cubs could not bring themselves to eat his body. Great Heart believed the mother tiger and her cubs were too weak and frail to break his skin, so he broke a branch from a tree and punctured it himself. As he began to bleed, the mother tiger and her cubs ate the flesh of Great Heart. At the same time, it began to rain flowers throughout the kingdom.

The five cubs became the first five fully ordained monks, and the mother tiger became the first fully ordained nun during Shakyamuni Buddha's time. Prince Great Heart became Shakyamuni Buddha himself.

My father told these stories to me before I moved to a monastery with my uncle when I became a monk at the age of six. Tears would come to my eyes when he recited them. When we learn about such great deeds and the Buddha's knowledge, we come to appreciate the great qualities of the Buddha's teaching, which have been transmitted through an unbroken lineage to the present day by the holy masters of India and Tibet.

Geshe Tsultim Gyeltsen, born in Tibet in 1927, studied for twenty-three years at Ganden Monastery where he earned the highest Geshe degree. In 1962 he completed his Tantric studies at Gyuto Tantric College. Gyeltsen has been teaching western students of Buddhism since 1963. In 1978 he founded Thubten Dhargye Ling, a center for Tibetan Buddhist studies and is the resident spiritual master.

A living being who in a previous life has not been one's parent
cannot be found, even by an omniscient mind.
All have cared for you, just as has your mother of this life.
Meditate on beings as having been your parents
and remember their infinite kindness.

HIS HOLINESS THE SEVENTH DALAI LAMA

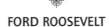

FORD ROOSEVELT

Buddhism and the Roosevelt Legacy

IN THE WINTER OF 1972 OR 1973, I WAS FORTUNATE TO BE IN THE AUDIENCE AT San Francisco College to hear a lecture by a Buddhist teacher, Alan Watts. As usual, he did not disappoint his eager and excited audience. In one exchange, Alan was asked where he came up with his histories of Mahayana Buddhism, the Middle Way. Quick as his laugh, he reached into his robe and pulled out a dog-eared copy of a small book, holding it up for all to see, and he proclaimed it a great book for all to read and learn the true origins of "The Middle Way." It was *The Secret Oral Teachings of Tibetan Buddhism* by Alexandra-David Neel. This was my first exposure to Tibetan Buddhism.

I had been an admirer of Alan's wonderful way of dispensing the Dharma from the moment I finished the first sentence of *The Way of Zen* in my college Eastern philosophy class. Coming from a structured Catholic upbringing, the sudden rush of this newly discovered "nature of reality" as explained by Alan Watts seemed to answer so many questions the nuns and priests could not.

While my Catholic education addressed a number of life's issues, it also left me wondering about many of the mysteries of life and obvious inequalities of the human condition. Perhaps being a "child of the '60s" added to my quest for spiritual comfort in that time of conflict. I was no doubt one of the thousands who heard Alan's message and those of other teachers during that special time. From Alan's books and references, I learned of the writings of D. T. Suzuki. The simplicity of the Zen experience had a strong appeal as an antidote to the overwhelming liturgy of the church with its myriad saints and sins.

From my first readings of Buddhist thought until now, I have never looked back from my belief that the teachings of the Buddha resonated with me in a way the Catholic Church had not been able to do. Within this structure, the legacy of being the grandson of Franklin and Eleanor Roosevelt lay dormant. It was not until my early forties that I began to find ways to examine the complexities of the Roosevelt legacy and how it might relate to my now deep adherence to the teachings of Buddha. My memories of my father, Elliott, and his relationship to his mother began to work their way back into my consciousness. He always told me what a wonderful woman she was, and how she was dedicated to peace throughout her life. He felt her deep and profound optimism. He, too, was one who always put forth a smile and a wish for something good to come of any situation in which he found himself, a trait he inherited from his mother. He told me about her vision of hope for humankind and how this carried her on through some of the most difficult times in her life.

The convergence of the message and legacy of my grandparents and my Buddhism happened quite by chance when I met, as fate would have it, a former Catholic priest, Jack Healy. Jack had been the executive director for Amnesty International for twelve or so years in the 1970s and 1980s. His nickname is "Mr. Human Rights" and he is a champion of the message of hope embodied in the United Nations Universal Declaration of Human Rights (UDHR). The U.N. General Assembly adopted this document on December 10, 1947 (see Appendix A for its complete text). It would be an understatement to say that my grandmother's role was anything less than significant in the drafting and passage of this historic document. She noted that chairing the committee that drafted the UDHR was the most important work of her entire life. Now, on December 10, 1996, I stood facing Mr. Human Rights, and he was asking me to stand up for my grandmother, for my legacy as a Roosevelt, and more important, for hope and human rights.

The message of Eleanor Roosevelt, one of hope and compassion for people around the world, is in perfect harmony with the message of Buddhism that I had struggled to define in my own life. It became as clear as the thirty articles in the UDHR. My "practice" and responsibility to the Roosevelt legacy is to work to spread the words of the UDHR, in places close to home, in schools and workplaces, in places so small they are not on maps. It is Eleanor's message—a clear call of hope and compassion detailed in this document.

My years of nonaffiliated practice came into clear focus, thanks again to Jack, through a meeting with His Holiness the Fourteenth Dalai Lama. My wife and children and I met with him for what seemed an eternity. He told us of his true affection for the work of my grandmother on the UDHR and how he still wears the watch sent to him by F.D.R. when he was a very young boy. As we parted and exchanged gifts, he asked for our help for Tibet and for human rights around the world. His words, in the following passage, continue to inspire me.

> *In today's highly interdependent world, individuals and nations can no longer resolve many of their problems by themselves. We need one another. We must therefore develop a sense of universal responsibility. It is our collective and individual responsibility to protect and nurture the global family, to support its weaker members, and to preserve and tend to the environment in which we all live.*

Once again, the Roosevelt legacy, the message of compassion, and the teachings of Buddha converge. What small part I play in spreading Eleanor's message and her work on the UDHR remains to be seen.

Ford Roosevelt is the managing director of Durlester Consulting, Inc., an executive search firm based in Southern California. Roosevelt is a board member of the World Committee on Disability based in Washington, D.C. and a member of the Family Committee of the Franklin and Eleanor Roosevelt Institute. Roosevelt is also active in the cause for Tibetan independence and serves on the board of directors for the Drepung Loseling Institute, a center for Tibetan Buddhist studies affiliated with Emory University in Atlanta, Georgia. Roosevelt and his wife, Marni, live in Sherman Oaks, California, and have three children.

The land mines in the ground
come from the land mines in our minds.
We must uproot both.

VENERABLE MAHA GHOSANANDA

❖

If you only have money to give,
then you may as well throw it
into the Bay of Bengal!

SISTER JESSE

❖

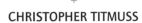

CHRISTOPHER TITMUSS

Awareness:
Springboard for Meditation and Politics

I CAN'T IMAGINE MEDITATION SEPARATE FROM CONCERN FOR THE WORLD. However, there is a difference between criticism and negativity, between constructive engagement and the dualism of "us and them." We do not need to regard one as the cause of the other. I do not believe that the self creates its own problems or that other people create our problems: problems arise simply because the conditions for them come into being. Nor do I believe that I have an exclusive inner truth or that some people have more of the truth than others. I do not consider myself to be a meditation teacher sometimes and a social activist at other times; I just focus on making a contribution to liberation through the resolution of the problems of humanity. Some problems appear to be located within the individual, and other problems within the structures that society has created for itself. But the mind and the structures remain inseparable from each other.

We need to dispense with the dualism of spirituality and politics, abandon all the associations that we have with these two areas, and look at things afresh. Then we may see that the two are already engaged. This shows itself in every word we say, every breath we take, and every moment of mindfulness. Engagement means a direct, active contribution toward the resolution of the problems of life.

The attitude of nonviolence plays an important role here, in both meditation and politics. The function of nonviolence comes from three specific standpoints. First is the moral injunction from which we might be prone to violence or retaliation, but as violence goes against our beliefs or values, we put a restraining order on our actions so as to maintain our commitment to nonviolence in the deeper sense.

Second is the depth of insight and realization that cannot give support to capital punishment or to inflicting violence intentionally on other human beings. At this point, nonviolence has gone beyond an act of will and has entered in a way of understanding.

Third is the approach of nonviolence as a useful and effective strategy. Killing and harming are gross tactics to deal with social, political, and economic problems. Violence, including throwing stones, firing bullets, laying land mines, or planting bombs, creates fear and mistrust. Strikes, demonstrations, noncooperation, negotiation, leaflets, and humor are more effective strategies and generate greater international support.

I was a monk with Venerable Maha Ghosananda, who exemplifies constructive nonviolence. He is Cambodian. He had seventeen relatives and all were murdered during the mid-1970s. Venerable Ghosananda left the monastery to work in the refugee camps of the Cambodians in Thailand. When the doors reopened, he went back to his country. Every May he walks through Cambodia to bring peace and justice. He went to the soldiers and said to them, "Lay down your rifles and kill the hate inside yourselves." He went to the parents of the soldiers and told them to tell their sons to lay down their rifles and kill the hate inside themselves. He went to the children of the soldiers and told them to tell their fathers, and so on. He has been nominated for the Nobel Peace Prize four times. We stood together on the steps of Capitol Hill in a U.N.–sponsored demonstration. Venerable Ghosananda told the media, "The land mines in the ground come from the land mines in our minds. We must uproot both."

I believe it is so important that the voices of constructive engagement take priority, or, as a former Palestinian freedom fighter told me, we must exchange words instead of bullets. We must keep faith with the strategies and approaches of constructive protest and engagement, no matter how difficult particular situations appear to be.

Three years ago I was asked to go to the West Bank and to take a select number of Israelis to spend three days there in Palestinian homes. This served as a springboard to other extended visits and to forming an organization, Face to Face. It aims to sustain contact with Palestinians and to lower the degree of fear, mistrust, and anger as a contribution to understanding. On a recent trip, the Israeli authorities had stopped entrance into the West Bank, so I went alone to the control point and walked across. I spent the day with my Palestinian friends and then brought back the report of what I had heard and seen to the Face to Face group. At that time there was a tremendous loss of faith in the peace process, and the result was Hamas terrorist bomb attacks. The people were despairing.

My work is dealing with the mutual understanding of each other and the tension of being an Israeli or a Palestinian. Meditation is not the reference point; rather it is communication and language. People must meet and get to know each other so that they see the common ground—their shared humanity, suffering, fear, insecurity. Then things start shifting. We all have far more in common than what separates us, and the communication has to be kept going at all cost, no matter how bad it may seem.

There are few things that I feel to be more important than working with anger. Anger harms ourselves as much as others. It is an ineffective way to achieve anything as it simply invites defensiveness or withdrawal from others, reinforcing dualism. There is no usefulness in any form of anger as a way of resolving human conflict. To imagine that we can just be angry toward one particular authority but full of kindness everywhere else is delusion. Any level of anger is unacceptable.

If we are not angry, then where will the energy come from, the adrenaline, that will motivate us to act? In fact, we need only the awareness of suffering; that should be enough to motivate anybody. When motivation is clear, then awareness is there. These two factors are vital, as in practicing loving-kindness, meditation, and equanimity. If anger is not being resolved inwardly, then we have to associate with those who maintain clear and constructive engagement. We're asking too much of people to be able to resolve their despair alone. I can't imagine anybody having wisdom or compassion without a community—a *sangha*—that gives ongoing support.

In 1990, several of us put together a school for about twenty children in Bodh Gaya. It is located in the middle of the state of Bihar, certainly the poorest place in India and maybe in South Asia. The school provides the poorest of the poor with education as a vital stepping-stone to awareness and change. We started off in a very modest way, but the school has now grown to some three hundred children. It is a true *sangha,* a vibrant community. There are Catholic nuns, Buddhist monks, Hindus, and Muslims all teaching in the school.

Our function as Westerners is to provide the financial resources to run the school and to ensure that the teachers are genuinely committed to interreligious awareness. We are not becoming colonial educationalists. In a talk to both Westerners and Asians there, Sister Jesse, a much-loved person, said it is not enough just to give money. We must make sacrifices and be prepared to offer something other than money. She said, "If you only have money to give, then you may as well throw it into the Bay of Bengal!" It was a dramatic statement. She was asking us to really extend ourselves.

I suspect that as we move into the new millennium, there will be a period of soul-searching among the affluent nations about their relationships to each other and to the rest of the world. Selfishness is the virus that pervades the human species. It destroys lives, communities, the welfare of societies, and Earth itself. Five years ago I had a meeting with one of my teachers, Achaan Buddhadasa. He spoke at length to me about selfishness. He commented rather wryly, "We won't destroy this world through ignorance but through being too clever. We have become too clever for our own good and too clever for everybody else's good." We must ask ourselves again and again what our priorities are. Is our daily life an honest statement of what matters? If not, we are wasting our existence on the trivial and immaterial. Our daily life states our values. There are no other criteria; we live by what we believe.

What do so many of the world's great heroes have in common? Meditation. They know the importance of the depths of meditation and awareness to contribute to loving-kindness. When we see the truth of who we are, then we know humanity is one, not fragmented. This vision influences our feelings, thoughts, and actions. We know that self and others are not separate. The war within has stopped.

Christopher Titmuss, a former Buddhist monk, teaches spiritual awakening and insight meditation retreats worldwide. He is the author of several books including *The Green Buddha, Light on Enlightenment,* and *An Awakened Life.* Titmuss is a member of the international advisory board of the Buddhist Peace Fellowship. In 1986 and 1992, he stood before the British Parliament for the Green Party. He is cofounder of Gaia House, an international retreat center in Devon, England. He is a parent and lives in Totnes, Devon.

Maitreya explained that he had been there all along,
but Asanga had been too self-centered to perceive his presence:
"I am Love, and you must have universal compassion
to be able to perceive Love."

FROM A BUDDHIST PARABLE

✴

JILL ANSELL

Asanga and the B Yard

THE GUYS FROM B YARD ENTERED THE CLASSROOM AS USUAL. BUT SOMEONE NEW was amongst the group and he stared at me with hungry eyes, as if I were a piece of meat in a butcher shop. My instant response was revulsion. I felt violated and I wanted him to leave immediately. Another inmate shouted to him, "Draper, what're you doing in here?" I was riveted. Draper. My mind was flooded with memories of Lena. Her dark skin, her warm lap, her loving words of comfort. Lena Draper. She was the earth, she was the ground, she was my surrogate mother. Lena worked for my family for many years and cared for me like a mother when my own mother was absent. I'll never forget the time we drove her home to her dark and dingy basement apartment. I had never been to a place like that. Standing in the prison classroom, memories raced through my mind, and I felt my heart turn in my chest. Revulsion and fear were transformed into warmth and compassion. I found a link to all Drapers as I recalled my warmth and love for Lena. The terrible prejudice and inequities African Americans have endured over time were etched in my consciousness early on. Through my love and compassion for Lena, I was instantly linked to the hearts of others exposed to such atrocities.

As an artist-in-residence at a state maximum-security prison, I am offered many opportunities to face my fears and prejudice. Each inmate has a story, and for each story there can be a turning of the heart. The most satisfying aspect of my work in the prison is accessing this compassion. Sharing the creative process with these men, many of whom have never received praise or finished a creative work, often brings them a sense of renewed hope and possibility. Many times I am challenged to break through the outer shell and reach a significant level of communication. Compassion and respect are the keys to this process.

My work in prisons supported my movement into Buddhism because I had become acutely aware of the suffering of sentient beings. When I heard His Holiness the Fourteenth Dalai Lama talk about the Four Noble Truths and the twelve links of dependent origination, I was deeply moved and profoundly relieved. It was then that I began to seriously study and practice Buddhism.

The practice of compassion prompted me to examine my experiences in ways I had never before done. A key component to the deepening of my insight was encountering the legendary story of the fourth-century saint, Asanga. For me, this story was the Aha! of insight into true compassion. At any moment, when I feel deficient in my attempt to generate compassion, I refer to it.

The Story of Asanga

Asanga, who grew dissatisfied with the state of Buddhism in his time, left his monastery while in his late twenties. He felt that even though it had only been eight hundred years since the time of the historical Shakyamuni Buddha, Buddhism was suffering from becoming overly formal, rote, and rigid. He made a personal resolution to retire into a cave and meditate ceaselessly until the future Maitreya Buddha appeared and revived the Buddhist teachings. For twelve years he prayed for a visionary encounter with the future Buddha, seemingly to no avail. Three times during this period, at three-year intervals, Asanga became discouraged and left his retreat, only to return later for further meditation.

At the end of the twelve-year period Asanga fell into total despair, suffered a complete loss of faith, and permanently departed from the cave. His life seemed to lack purpose and meaning, and his hope for a vision of Maitreya had vanished. As he wandered aimlessly, he came upon an old dog that had been severely injured. Her hindquarters had a large, festering sore that was teeming with maggots. Asanga took interest in the suffering animal and resolved to heal her. As he began to remove the maggots, he realized that they would be crushed and killed if he were to pick them off with his fingers. With this in mind, he cut a strip of flesh from his thigh to serve as their resting and feeding ground. Since he had resolved not to injure the maggots, he stretched out his tongue onto the wound to entice them to crawl onto it so he could transfer them to his severed flesh.

As he was doing this an explosion of light flashed in front of him, and when he looked up he found Maitreya standing before him. He asked the Buddha why he had taken so many years to appear. Maitreya explained that he had been there all along, but Asanga had been too self-centered to perceive his presence. "I am Love, and you must have universal compassion to be able to perceive Love. If you don't believe me, take me to the people and see what happens." Placing Maitreya on his shoulder, Asanga walked to town. Sadly, the townspeople perceived Maitreya as the sick, old dog, thought Asanga was mad, and drove him out of town.

Not only does this story point to the deep level of compassion required for the process of mind transformation, it also serves to remind me about how my projections and fears block my practice of compassion. Maintaining faith and constantly remembering Asanga's exquisite vision—despite the fact that it is not shared by many—links me to all of life. When I recall this story as I enter the prison gate, I go about the day's work with a more enlightened perspective. Therein lies the daily task of transforming one's mind into a vehicle of love. Thank you, Asanga. And thanks to my dear Venerable Teacher, Geshe Tsultim Gyeltsen, whose thorough teachings lead me to the heart of the Dharma.

Jill Ansell is an artist and arts educator whose paintings have been exhibited and published widely. Through her work as an artist-in-residence, she has touched the lives of many inmates at the state prisons in California. She currently resides in Los Angeles.

Practice poses the question, "What is This?"
and by doing so, reminds us that that which we seek
is directly in front of us.

DIANE RIZZETTO

❀

✦

DIANE RIZZETTO

Hide and Seek

ONCE, LONG AGO, THERE WAS A KING OF GREAT WEALTH AND LEARNING WHO ruled a vast kingdom. He busied himself by studying all that was made available to him: music, art, philosophy, magic. His reputation grew wide, and he was known as the most learned king around. As a way of keeping his thirst for knowledge quenched, the king would invite scholars from all over his kingdom to dine with him and engage in discussion on all sorts of topics. Nevertheless, he would soon tire of meeting with the same people, and his attendants' greatest challenge became finding individuals who could keep the king's intellect satiated.

Not far from the king's castle lived a young boy whose wisdom was known by many of the people. News of him came to the king's assistant and he suggested to the king that he invite the young boy to one of his dinners. The king replied, "But who is this boy? Surely he is too young to engage in any worthy discourse. With whom has he studied and what are his credentials?" "None, my Lord," answered his attendant. "I only know that all who know of him attest to his great wisdom."

Out of curiosity the king invited the boy to dinner and soon after they feasted, the king was ready to engage in discourse. But the boy wasn't interested in talking. Rather, he suggested, "Let's play hide and seek!" The king, thinking he would humor the boy for a while, agreed but suggested that since he was skilled in magic that the boy should hide first. But the boy would have no part of it and insisted that the king hide first. So with a wave of the hand, the king disappeared into another realm. The boy let out a sigh, as only children can do, and protested, "That's no fun. How can we play if you're in another world?" So the king materialized again and said, "Okay, let's see what you can do." With the blink of an eye, the boy disappeared, leaping deep into the heart of the king. The king looked everywhere, searching for the boy. Finally the boy yelled out, "Here I am!" but the king didn't hear. Each time the king called for another hint, the boy yelled louder but the king never heard. Finally, the king said, "I give up. Please show yourself." With another blink of the eye, the boy reappeared and the king said, "With all my great knowledge I could not find out. Where were you?" The boy answered, "I was in your heart all the time. If you do not look into your own heart first, then you will never find what you seek."

Learning how to look into our hearts, to find what prevents us from seeing, is much of what a life of practice is about. We're in a very confusing situation. On one hand we desperately seek some understanding of our distress, our hurts, our doubts, our fears, and our pains; but on the other hand, we actively hide from that which leads us to understanding. Most of us are like the king in the story. We look everywhere but in the most obvious place for the source of our contentment, playing a game of hide and seek. When we're "it," we usually skip the most obvious places and search everywhere else. Practice poses the question, "What is This?" and by doing so, it reminds us that that which we seek is directly in front of us. But who among us understands this without a great deal of prodding? Not many. If we ever want to understand in a very clear way the course of our suffering, we must be willing to come out of hiding and slowly come face to face with ourselves. Like the king, we are experts at hiding—even magicians of sorts. We can hide in our work, becoming too busy to stop and reflect, to listen, to just sit still. Even after meditating for years, we can become too busy to do *zazen;* too busy to come to the center; too busy to come to *sesshin;* too busy for waking up.

Of course, there is nothing wrong with being busy. We all have times in our lives when we quickly move from one activity to the next. But especially at those times, we can stop and ask some important questions. Why am I doing this? Who am I serving? What is my intention? Has doing become an avoidance of experiencing? Does busy (especially if it's a "worthy" busy) keep us hidden from experiencing what is in our hearts? Maybe our hiding place is behind an aura of self-sufficiency—not allowing ourselves to depend on someone else for fear we may be rejected, abandoned, hurt. Perhaps we duck behind some type of authority—a person, a teacher, a mentor, a boss—so that we don't have to chance making the wrong decision, a decision that may make us feel rejected or inadequate. There is no shortage of places to hide. If we're not careful, we can even hide in a Zen practice by retreating into altered states of mind that bring us temporary relief from our pain, mistaking the altered state for enlightenment. For whatever reason we hide, we cannot escape the truth of our experience. To hide from it, we hide from ourselves. When we hide from ourselves, we lose ourselves. So the aim of our Zen practice is to bring us out of hiding to meet ourselves.

So how do we come out of hiding? In truth, there is no real hiding place. We cannot escape what we are, but like the king in the story, we can have a deaf ear. The voice that can jolt us awake is soft and hardly audible at times. It's easy to ignore it or for it to be drowned out by the din. If we're fortunate, and if we're willing to listen, we can find a teacher in any event, in any person, and in any moment. And when we can just be there in that experience, even for only a second or two, we've come out of hiding. This is easy to say, for sure, but not so easily done. Because, like the king, the place we want to look is where we already are.

We must be coaxed and prodded, by the voice that is sometimes

97

inside us and sometimes outside us. We all have that voice. It's what brings about the seeking to begin with. Sometimes the voice is very tiny; sometimes it's very loud. But always, it urges us to ask questions. What is this? What is happening? Who am I, in this very moment?

Diane Rizzetto was born in Boston, Massachusetts, married at a young age, and had three children. In 1978 she moved to California and soon afterward began studying with Sojun Mel Weitsman at the Berkeley Zen Center. After several years there, she began studying with Charlotte Joko Beck of the Zen Center of San Diego. Rizzetto received Dharma transmission from Joko in 1994 and was installed as teacher and abbot of the Bay Zen Center. In addition to her Zen teaching, Rizzetto works as a learning therapist and spends time with her husband and four grandchildren.

Chikudo: The Bamboo Way
(To Masakazu Yoshizawa)

My teacher sits beside me,
Holding his *shakuhachi* like an oar.
Blow as though you were
a fisherman rolling a boat.
He walks the rhythm, hums
the tune. I see myself alone,
small waves rocking my boat
like a cradle. I stop and wait.

He explains: each *note, each phrase*
has a shape. Like a leaf.
With thumb and finger he makes
the movement, narrow, then wider
at the top, he brings it to a close.
I want to see this in your sound:
two falling leaves and a root.

He reminds me: You *have nowhere*
To go; you are in the mountains.
I am on the bike, concentrating

on every rock and curve, braking
before I fall. I ask someone the way
to Sturtevant Falls. *You're almost there.*
When I see a cascade at the end
of the path I think I am there.
This is the way it is, just to say
I've arrived, somewhere.

I am learning to play *chikudo:*
The bamboo way, with my legs
tucked under my bottom and a pillow
to cushion my aging knees. I think
of those old men on stage at Koyasan Hall
entranced by their own sound,
no sheet music, eyes closed as in *zazen,*
oblivious to the occasional cough,
the swish of fans.

CAROL LEM

❖

CAROL LEM

Suizen: Blowing Meditation

THE *SHAKUHACHI,* OR JAPANESE BAMBOO FLUTE, CAME INTO MY LIFE IN THE 1960s, at exactly the right moment. I was in my twenties, and all around me seeds of rebellion were sprouting questions about where I was going, where I had been. Amidst the political, societal, and familial clamor, I was searching for a way out, or a way in—inside myself. And though I did not realize it then, I was searching for a sound. As a child, I studied piano with my Aunt Ethel; as a teenager I played a cornet in the Chinese Drum and Bugle Corps—both under the watchful eyes of my parents. The Western flute I chose for myself was a response to a growing love for Debussy and things solitary. But it wasn't until I heard a record of *honkyoku* (meditation pieces for the *shakuhachi*) that something else called to me. The something else led me to Sensei Wakita and his group Baido-Kai, who performed once a year at Koyasan Hall in Little Tokyo. But after eight years or so of lessons and performances, that something else eluded me, and I respectfully placed my *shakuhachi* in the closet for fifteen years.

At the tender age of forty-six, finding myself once again in a spiritual crisis, I spotted a few Japanese students in the English class I was teaching at East Los Angeles College and asked, "Does anyone know of a *shakuhachi* teacher?" It just so happened that one woman did, the man who tuned her piano. What synchronicity! Not only did he live in my neighborhood,

Temple City, but he also had inherited many of Sensei Wakita's flutes and much of his sheet music; he was good friends with his daughter, Kayoko, whose house I used to visit for my weekly lessons. At my first lesson with Masakazu Yoshizawa, he wanted to hear how I played *Rokudan*. After a few passages, he stopped me and sighed, "You can play the notes okay, but your playing is mechanical." He proceeded to draw a map of techniques to bring out the sound of the bamboo, that sound that had once eluded me. Hence began *chikudo,* the bamboo way, which continues to this day.

Living the bamboo way is a devotion to a sound. To become that sound is to reach a high level of spiritual development, as in Basho's teaching, "Learn about the pine from the pine, learn about the bamboo from the bamboo." Learn about yourself from yourself with the bamboo flute as your practice. Just as *zazen* means sitting meditation, *suizen* means blowing meditation. Practice now is not those tedious mechanical scales I played in my aunt's living room, but a way of playing them. As Sensei Yoshizawa is always reminding me, "It's not what you play, it's how you play it." "Just playing slowly is not meditation. It's also playing fast." But as in all spiritual practices, the struggle is to nurture a certain state of mind. For after the techniques are mastered, then what? What is that difference between the student's sound and that of Katsuya Yokoyama? How do you teach that? That's the mystery.

The relationship between teacher *(sensei)* and student is reflected in the way they sit with each other during the lesson. Traditionally, as was the case with Mr. Wakita and still is in Japan, the student sits opposite the teacher, the space between them, the unshared space, symbolizing that one is above the other. So when Masakazu Yoshizawa, or Masa, came to my home for my first lesson, I set up the chairs with the music stand between us. The first thing he did was to place my chair next to his, saying only, "It's easier to read the music together." Only later did I learn that his departure from traditional custom was a tribute to the relationship between teacher and student; we were participating in a shared teaching and learning experience. He is a demanding instructor because he treats his students as professionals. Respect for musical composition and interpretation is at the core of his teaching. He is concerned with honoring the music, not the teacher. Yet each of us pays the highest honor to Masa by practicing well.

Like Japanese poetry, *shakuhachi* music, in particular *honkyoku*, is a reflection of nature, so Masa's teaching focuses on shaping the sound to the music's content. For example, in *Tsuru no Sugomori (Nesting Cranes)*, the sound of cranes, which is close to a fluttering sound, is created by a technique called *koro koro*, a precise way of moving your fingers. The challenge is to create this subtle pattern of sounds without fluttering the fingers. He told me to practice this while visualizing a nesting crane, before playing the whole piece. Imaging a crane was not easy, so I looked it up in the dictionary for the picture. I incorporated the crane into my poetry and listened to *shakuhachi* masters like Goro Yamaguchi, to immerse myself in imagery and sound. One Sunday, while going through the travel section of the newspaper, I came upon a misty photograph of a place in Japan where people go just to see cranes. I cut it out, hoping one day to paint it. As Basho might say, "Be the crane by going to the crane." Short of going to Japan, painting the cranes and blowing their sound are ways of going to the crane.

Another birdlike sound, *tamane*, is created by placing the tip of your tongue on the roof of your mouth, right behind your front teeth, then blowing. Since this was an impossible task in the beginning, he told me to practice making the fluttering sound without the flute. So I'd walk around the house fluttering my tongue. I fluttered my tongue while cooking and putting the dishes away. I fluttered my tongue in the shower while chanting a sound which had the effect of *OM*. Once this began to feel natural, I then played the note using *tamane*, which took me to a place I hadn't been before. Perhaps because more air is used, or so it seems for the beginner, a slight light-headedness created an airy feeling close to a high in meditation. While practicing *Tsuru no Sugomori* and *Sanya (Three Valleys)*, I continue to struggle with getting *koro koro* and *tamane* right. If sound reflects content, then this may be appropriate. In a piece like *Sanya*, for example, the three valleys refer to three high-pitched melodies or echoing sounds, or the three high points in the struggle toward enlightenment.

Masa is constantly reminding me that in my effort to get it right, I risk losing the mood and the music. This is especially crucial in rhythmic passages, as in ensemble pieces with *koto* and *shamisen* in which just playing the notes right is not enough. I often find myself so concerned with moving my fingers correctly, staying on pitch and timing, that my playing sounds like a bunch of notes. "You're not listening to yourself!" is a refrain I've heard over the years. Masa suggests that I imagine my spirit leaving my body and listening to me play, like someone is playing me, and I am the flute.

Masa says, "It's never the same," meaning you never play the same piece in the same way, as in Heraclitus's statement, "You never step in the same water twice." All depends on your mood, the atmosphere around you, and your relationship to the piece at that moment. In this way, the *shakuhachi* is a mirror of the player's soul. As a tool of meditation, then, it helps me to look within. If I feel somewhat scattered or exhausted by the day's events, my playing will reflect that. So I will blow *ro,* low D, for ten minutes. When I find thoughts entering my mind, I let them fall away like leaves by bringing my attention back to my blowing until I hear my sound (my soul) clarify itself. After centering, I am ready to practice. Masa calls this "relaxed attention." As in *zazen,* where the posture itself is the meditation, so in *suizen.* Whether sitting in a chair or on the floor, you slowly raise the *shakuhachi* from your lap to your lips, eyes cast slightly down, back straight—this posture triggers a state of meditation, a readiness to begin playing.

That the Japanese bamboo flute called to me in a way that the Western flute didn't has to do with these techniques that merge *you,* whoever that *you* is or is becoming, with the bamboo. I remember when Masa was teaching me *komibuki,* a breathing technique in which an unrefined vibrato is created by pumping the diaphragm. He first demonstrated this without the *shakuhachi* by making a *hoo, hoo, hoo* sound as his stomach bounced up and down. He then gave me a piece to try: *Sagariha (Falling Leaves).* As after doing *koro koro* for the first time, I felt a little light-headed, which helped me imagine the staccato falling of leaves moved by the wind. After practicing this technique in other pieces, it began to sound natural.

Indeed, there are times when I'm doing *komibuki* that I feel like a windswept tree, or like falling leaves. When these moments come and my entire being resonates through the bamboo, the *shakuhachi* is a projection of self. And the *you* who walked into the practice room an hour before is not the *you* blowing *Sagariba*. In fact, there is no *you*. There is only the practice room *(dojo)*, the *shakuhachi*, and the playing. In these rare moments my spirit has left the body and someone or something is playing me. That something else that called to me in my twenties, this sound that Masa is teaching me to keep inside my life, is *chikudo*, the bamboo way.

Carol Lem has studied the bamboo flute *(shakuhachi)* with Masakazu Yoshizawa for ten years. Her other practice is writing poetry. She has published poems in *Asian Pacific American Journal, Blue Mesa Review, Chrysalis, Hawaii Pacific Review, Luna, Rattle, The Seattle Review,* and others. She also teaches creative writing, literature, and composition at East Los Angeles College. Her home page at is www.members. aol.com/clem64079/peddlerpress.

Listening carefully to the tone, where or how does it move and in which direction? When you discover the answer, the tone itself will reveal many directions. Do not try to control it yourself!

MIYAJIMA SENSEI

✦

✦

MASAKAZU YOSHIZAWA

My Music, My Destiny

THE MOUNTAINS AND RIVERS, THE SOUNDS OF DRUMS AND FLUTES AT FESTIVALS
and celebrations, were all part of my environment when I was growing up.
These were not music, but rather the sounds of my village, where boys usually practiced *kendo* (Japanese fencing) and those pursuing music were not
taken seriously. Much of my joy, however, was in visiting the town music
store and perusing scores and admiring instruments. I chose the clarinet
during middle school and practiced on my own, becoming a self-taught
player. Part of my academic training was in Western music, but much of
the Western influence came from television or radio. In retrospect, some
of my best instructors of Western music imparted a rather disciplined, traditionally Japanese style of instruction.

During my high school years, Kurano Sensei came to teach at our
school. Thus began my basic training—the most important part of my
musical life. The concept of basic training may sound simple, yet what is
basic training? It includes the study of pitch or intonation, rhythm, and
tone quality. Do we really understand in our hearts what these elements
are? To master them is a challenge. Once we master them, are we playing
them in our hearts? Are we singing them in our hearts? These questions
and reminders were drilled into me by Kurano Sensei. About this time, a
friend commented on how difficult it was to play the *shakuhachi*—even to

make a sound. I thought about it for a moment and decided that that should not be, and I promptly began practicing the *shakuhachi*. Most of my practice, however, was in private: hidden in corners of trains or unnoticed areas of the school. I was quite aware that, at the time, traditional instruments and music were ridiculed. The focus was on Western music.

I eventually chose the clarinet as my main instrument and pursued my studies with Miyajima Sensei. He showed me another dimension of the philosophy of music. He asked, "Listening carefully to the tone, where or how does it move and in which direction? When you discover the answer, the tone itself will reveal many directions. Do not try to control it yourself!" Miyajima Sensei's lessons were out of the ordinary. There were never critical suggestions, technical demonstrations, or any kind of advice. I decided to visit his home for further study. He welcomed me and we embarked on hours of discussions about music and its philosophy. In time, my life was filled with performances and concerts of Western music. One day, while preparing for a concert, Miyajima Sensei asked me, "What is important in a concert?" I replied, "Musical sensitivity, talent, and technique." His immediate response was "Intonation, rhythm, and tone quality." After stressing the basics he added, "Then, musicianship and talent."

In 1976, I came to the United States and continued as a clarinetist. But one day I was called to assist in the musical *Teahouse of the August Moon*. The director suggested that since I was Japanese it was only natural for me to perform on the Japanese flute. I soon returned to Japan to reunite with the *shakuhachi* and took lessons. Even when I was an inexperienced *shakuhachi* player, this instrument seemed very natural for me. We were like kindred souls connecting. It is interesting for me to realize that studying the clarinet always required "playing well." The *shakuhachi*, on the other hand, has no such requirement. One is not conscious of playing well but is aware of following the tone, trying to become at one with that tone.

One year, Yamato Sensei came from Japan, and I had the opportunity to study the traditional technique of the Kinko School. Traditional Japanese lessons consist of imitating the teacher. The style has continued for decades. While I was impressed with Yamato Sensei's technique and tone, I knew in my heart how I wished to relate to the *shakuhachi*. I had studied with Western-trained music teachers but they were Japanese. I must assume that their Japanese identity conveyed to me a traditional philosophy about music even though they were teaching Western instruments.

I also had the pleasure of studying with Katada Sensei (National Living Treasure of Japan) Kabuki percussion or Hayashi music. A traditionally disciplined instructor, the student and he sat facing one another, and the teaching was done orally. He departed from traditional percussionists who claimed that the concept of *Ma,* a kind of unmeasured space, cannot be understood or felt by Westerners. Katada Sensei responded that *Ma* could indeed be measured and conducted in the Western manner. It is not a matter of cultural identity. Simply put, Katada Sensei stated, "It is *accelerando* and *ritardando* in extreme! Important, too, is understanding the composition well, knowing the history and culture of the period, and possessing a sixth sense."

I have studied both Western and Japanese traditional music and pursued the truth of music most of my life. I may never reach that goal, but I must continue just the same. I am certain of one thing: as I bridge the two, they become more and more an integral part of my life and music.

Masakazu Yoshizawa is a composer and an active studio musician for woodwinds, Japanese bamboo flute *(shakuhachi),* and percussion. Among his soundtrack recordings are *Jurassic Park, The Joy Luck Club,* and *Lost World.* His CDs include *Kyori, Sorin, Wakyo,* and *Zen Garden.* His worldwide tours, which include performances with his group, Kokin Gumi, are nationally televised in Japan.

In meditation we give the mind a shining model and study it
very carefully every morning and every evening until it is printed on
our hearts. Then, throughout the rest of the day,
we go along chipping away at everything that is not Self.
It takes many years, but in the end, the great mystics
of all religions tell us, every bit of anger, fear, and
greed can be removed from our consciousness,
so that our whole life becomes a flawless work of art.

SRI EKNATH EASWARAN

✦

ROBERT NICHOLS

Life As a Work of Art

MY HEART'S RESPONSE TO BEAUTY HAS NEVER BEEN ENTIRELY PEACEFUL. WHEN I sit in a redwood grove, listening to children's voices vanish into silence, there is peace but there is also restlessness, a disquiet beneath the surface. It's not enough to listen and see. In the deepest part of my heart, the beauty is a call that urges response, like a mother answering her calling child. Not to respond, not to return the gift, would somehow be a betrayal, a turning away from who we are and from where we have come.

An artist feels that call, responds to it, accepts the restlessness it brings, and works passionately toward the peace that comes from answering. Listening, watching, feeling are never an end in themselves. A ravishing piece of music, the movement of a dancer, a quiet moment when death and birth are near—these are not experiences but invitations to a passionate conversation. They are an intimate romance which promises a beautiful child: a work of art.

For years, as a dancer and choreographer, I pursued this romance, but I became gradually aware of a deeper restlessness, a more insistent call that was not being answered. I felt painfully the limitations of my art. I tried to expand my work, taking on bigger themes, creating new works with commissioned music and involving fine art. But the call seemed to be about so much more than these little things.

My equation was no longer working. Even when a work was finished, I felt no peace, no sense of completion. One day I drove to the beach and spent a long time walking, reading, ruminating. I remember tossing a few stones into the ocean and feeling that my work would be swallowed up just as completely, without ever truly responding to this inner call.

At about that time, I met Sri Eknath Easwaran for the first time and heard him speak. There was a beauty about him and what he said, a kind of majesty about his bearing, his words, his glance. He seemed to me like a great artist: confident, whole, generous, yet with his eyes fixed on a distant, uncompromising goal. There was utter peace but also a burning restlessness that touched my heart and made me long for great things. He seemed to be both the ideal response to the call, and the call itself.

His teachings appealed to me: that the supreme goal is possible, that all traditions have produced people that reached it, that you could be devoted to Buddha, Christ, Sri Krishna without conflict. But one particular teaching seemed directed specifically to my yearning. It became my motto and inspiration: "You can make your entire life a work of art." The words you speak, the work you do, the love you give, even your food and recreation can all become a radiant expression of beauty, responses to the call. In fact, such a life is the only perfect response, the only act of creation, which brings real peace.

To my intellect, this teaching seemed paradoxical. To my heart, it was urgent and immediate. With much meditation and struggle, the image has become clearer. The only response that we can hope to make to the great Beauty, the only one that will bring the peace of true creation, is the response that Beauty has already created in our heart: love, patience, compassion. By revealing it, we will give beauty to beauty, and participate in the immortal process.

In this process, I have found fulfillment as an artist and moments of profound peace, as well as immense restlessness. With each step, the call is more demanding, and what I have to give seems more insignificant. And yet, the mystery and beauty of spiritual life continues to grow. As I struggle to love, to give, to create in response to the call, there come moments when beauty is revealed; not beauty I have created, but primeval beauty, immense and tiny, eternal and fleeting. I love in spite of myself, beyond myself. Where they come from I do not know, but I do know that this beauty is truly within me and that I will listen again—eagerly, impatiently—for the next call that will challenge me to respond.

Robert Nichols grew up in Berkeley, California. In his career as a ballet dancer he performed with the Chicago City Ballet, the Oakland Ballet, Berkeley Ballet Theater, and other small companies around California and the United States. In 1985 he became a student of Sri Eknath Easwaran and joined the Blue Mountain Center of Meditation, where he lives and works today.

God is Magic.
God lives in the heart.
We can't see Him because our eyes
don't see inside ourselves.
But if you try to see inside yourself,
then you can see Him.
He is not air, but air is a part of Him.
He is not water, but water is a part of Him.
He is not earth, but earth is a part of Him.
Just like your nose is not you,
but is a part of you.

BABA HARI DASS

BABA HARI DASS

God Is Peace

ASPIRANTS TO GOD ATTAIN THE VERY GOD THEY FORM IN THEIR MINDS. IF THEY think God is light, God appears as light. If they think God is sound, God appears as sound. If they think God has a human form, God appears in human form. Actually, all these appearances of God are the illusions of the mind, because God is beyond name and form. He is everything and nothing. But the illusion is true to the person who sees it, and it brings a conviction of truth.

It's easy to worship a form of God because we can see it and feel it. This can be a good method of worship, but after reaching a higher state of mind, the name and form of God disappear. In worshipping God with form, we attain God according to our vision of Him. But God is beyond form, and the illusion will eventually take us to the real God.

God to me is inner peace. When the mind is freed from the outer turmoil of the world, it becomes peaceful. In that peaceful state of mind, God's love can be experienced. Ultimately, this love has no explanation, but rather is a pure state of mind.

When I was six years old I started feeling trapped in the world. The sky and earth became a box for me and I began to feel closed inside. My mind had imprisoned itself—but projected a box in the outer world. In that agitated state of mind, a strong desire to leave developed. But to leave what?

After I knocked on several doors to find the answer, it came from inside: Leave all those things that disturb the peace. When the mind is in peace, that is internal existence—and that is God. That is why I use the term *peace* to explain God. Peace is not a dual state but an ever-existing reality.

The essence of my teaching is to understand ourselves. We best go about this goal by first realizing that the outer world is nothing more than a projection of our inner lives. We create it by our egos, out attachments, and our desires. If something appears bad or wrong in the world, its cause is inside us, not in the outer world. If we can truly understand this cause and effect, then we can let go of egos, attachments, and desires, thus setting the stage to experience God's love.

Ultimately, we are all capable of understanding this simple truth: Peace can indeed be found in this world—and God is peace. The more our minds are involved in the outer things of the world, the less we understand ourselves and the less we experience God.

As long as we have the ego of being a "doer," we can't be completely free. Diving for pearls is easy, but when we have pearls we also develop the fear of losing them. There is no peace in pearls, so diving for God is better, although harder.

Attachment to the world (my house, my garden, my son, my daughter) and the ego that "I am the doer" (doctor, lawyer, minister, businessperson, yogi) chains us so tightly that we don't want to lose our attachments, even if we know that when we lose them we will attain eternal peace. We want to remain in the pain of "I am the doer."

Ego is important for achieving success in the world, but if directed this way it can be a great obstacle to attaining real peace. We are social beings; we can't live without a society. But to move in society we need existence, or ego, which brings us back again to the question: How can we find peace? If we understand that the world is unreal and is only a projection of our egos, if we act in the world only as we perform our duties, then there is peace everywhere for us.

I cultivated my inner peace and relationship with God by fighting within myself, by my inner successes and defeats. This peace, or experience of God, now separates the two worlds for me; the outer world is still projected, but without the attachment that gives it a reality. An analogy would be a man who decides to sell his new car—the car can still be beautiful without belonging to him.

If we are to create a peaceful world in the future we must begin with the experience of inner peace, the experience of God. God is not somewhere else; we are God. We are God and we are in God. It's simply a matter of acceptance. Accept yourself, accept others, and accept the world. When you do, pain will still come, just like pleasure. Hate will come, just like love. And when both are accepted, unaffected by the peaceful mind—there will be peace on earth.

Baba Hari Dass is a silent monk who has not spoken since 1952 and communicates by writing on a small chalkboard. He is first and foremost a master yogi, having practiced the disciplines of yoga from childhood. He is also an accomplished author, teacher, builder, philosopher, sculptor, and proponent of Ayurveda (the ancient Indian system of health and healing). Under his direction, the California-based Hanuman Fellowship was formed in 1974.

Even if you are considered to be the most sinful of all sinners,
when you are situated in the boat of transcendental knowledge
you will be able to cross over the ocean of miseries.

BHAGAVAD GITA

✳

BOB COHEN

Saint or Sinner?

IN 1970, I READ THE FOLLOWING VERSE FROM THE FOURTH CHAPTER OF THE
Bhagavad Gita, and it changed my life. It reads, "Even if you are considered
to be the most sinful of all sinners, when you are situated in the boat of transcendental knowledge you will be able to cross over the ocean of miseries"
(BG 4.36). At the time, I was a junior majoring in science at Rensselaer
Polytechnic Institute, taking a survey course on oriental philosophies. The
only studies of real interest to me were philosophy and sociology. I had a
long-standing attraction to India, and yet knew very few Indians, had not
traveled there, and had read few books about Indian philosophy or culture.
When the Nehru suits came out, I was twelve or thirteen years old and could
not rest until I had one. I took the course seriously (much more so than
chemistry or physics) and really tried to grasp the *Gita,* especially this verse,
which stuck in my mind. I asked my professor to explain it. I was mystified
by the idea that one could be a sinner and a saint at the same time. My black-
and-white '60s view of the world was showing. The professor responded that
it was "intuitively obvious"; in other words, you can only understand
through intuition, not logical explanation.

Several years earlier I had visited Greenwich Village regularly, just to
observe. During one such sojourn I saw Hare Krishna devotees singing and
dancing. I was intrigued, amazed, and confused. Were they exhibitionists

or renunciates? They wore simple Indian dress and mismatched socks. The men had shaved heads and ponytails and clay marks on their bodies, and they looked blissful while chanting. I stared and watched and listened. I eventually learned the words and chanted to myself: Hare Krishna, Hare Krishna, Krishna Krishna, Hare Hare; Hare Rama, Hare Rama, Rama Rama, Hare Hare. I had no idea of the meaning, but the chanting was pleasurable.

Meanwhile, I had applied to the Peace Corps and put India as my first choice of country. One year later, shortly before graduation, I was accepted. I had actually forgotten I had applied and had become engaged to my wife. She knew nothing about India, nor much about my long-standing and keen interest in it. I was torn apart. Do I leave my love and go on my adventure, or stay and preserve my dear and wonderful relationship? Fortunately for me, Bhakti (Barbara then) decided for me. "Go and I will wait. You will never be satisfied if you do not have your adventure." Her wisdom then, as now, is profound.

Shortly after graduation I was on a thirty-two-hour plane ride to New Delhi. After a few weeks' training there, the Peace Corps sent me off for a weekend jaunt on my own to test my burgeoning language and cultural skills. Arriving in Thanesur, about 100 miles north of New Delhi, I found out that the town is the train station for Kuruksetra, the very battlefield where the *Gita* was spoken. There I was standing on the actual *Gita* battlefield, preserved as a memorial. I inquired of the local population if they chanted; I wanted to know if the chant was a Western customization or a native tradition. As with many things in India I rarely got a straight answer. My limited Hindu and their Queen's English were obstacles to our communication, but more so was my lack of understanding of the local theological position. The *Gita* I read was a monotheistic poem. The Hinduism I met was a polytheistic, pantheistic hodge-podge. Without understanding this difference I could not communicate my fundamental question as to the validity of chanting Hare Krishna.

After the better part of a year, I had not yet satisfied my initial curiosity about India; I found the local religion to be akin to the United States' televised evangelism. Hence, I traveled to other areas seeking to quench my curious thirst. During a visit to Calcutta, I spotted a poster for a Hare Krishna festival happening just then, so I jumped a trolley to the designated place. I heard a talk by Giriraja Swami, a disciple of A. C. Bhaktivedanta Swami (also known as Prabhupada) that struck a chord. He described how the Indian masses were attracted to the material culture of the West, which the followers of Prabhupada rejected. He was dressed in native Bengali clothes and the Bengalis were dressed in Western suits and ties. My curiosity was piqued. I began to visit the Hare Krishna Center whenever I was in Calcutta. The place had an intense strangeness, with the chanting devotees, the deities, and the musky incense.

In February 1972, on one of my now regular visits to Calcutta, I came across a Hare Krishna devotee who invited me to a festival in Mayapur on the bank of the Ganges, about 60 miles north. The Hare Krishnas had recently bought some land at an historic holy place. Since I was on break from my Peace Corps teaching, I gladly went. I found Mayapur to be beautiful with its rice paddies, small villages, misty mornings, and traditional *bhajans* (devotional chanting) in the villages. The Hare Krishna land was undeveloped, with just a hut for Prabhupada, a women's tent, a men's tent, and a colorful tent for a temporary temple. I was the only person at the site who was not a follower of Prabhupada or a native of the area. After a day or so, Prabhupada's secretary noticed me and asked if I would like to meet Prabhupada. I was definitely interested, having already met him briefly in Calcutta, and having been struck by his humble yet commanding demeanor, his detached yet concerned air.

I walked into his hut. Prabhupada asked, "Do you have any questions?" I did not know any Sanskrit, not a word, and that was obvious. Yet, the very first verse Prabhupada quoted to me was that same verse that had mystified me in college, BG 4.36. He only quoted the Sanskrit but assumed I knew the English, which I did. This was the only verse in the *Gita* I knew. Even though this verse is not one of the more profound statements of the *Gita*, he obviously felt it was the right one for that moment. Following my intuition had led me to my spiritual master and signaled me to listen carefully to his words.

Through the years, my understanding of that verse has deepened. My vision subsequently transformed from my youthful black-and-white categorization of folks to my trying to see the higher aspirations within everyone, saint and sinner alike. Prabhupada's embodiment of the verse, and the words of the verse itself, continue to inspire and uplift me.

Bob Cohen is an environmental consultant specializing in groundwater issues and a trainer for the Federal Environmental Protection Agency. Since serving in the Peace Corps in India from 1971 to 1972, Cohen has been a member of the Hare Krishna Movement. In the Krishna Conscious Society, he focuses on higher education. A book about his experiences in India has been translated into thirty-seven languages. Cohen has been married twenty-eight happy years and has two children.

If a man has compassion, he is Buddha,
Without compassion, he is Lord of Death.

With compassion, the root of Dharma is planted,
Without compassion, the root of Dharma is rotten.

One with compassion is kind even when angry,
One without compassion kills even as he smiles.

For one with compassion, even enemies turn into friends,
Without compassion, even friends turn into enemies.

With compassion, one has all Dharmas,
Without compassion, one has no Dharma at all.

With compassion, one is a true Buddhist,
Without compassion, one is worse than profane.

Even meditating on voidness, one needs compassion as its essence.
A Dharma practitioner must have a compassionate nature.

Great compassion is like a wish-fulfilling gem.
Great compassion fulfills the hopes of self and others.

Therefore, all of you, renunciates and householders,
Cultivate compassion and you will achieve Buddhahood.

SHABKAR

MATTHIEU RICARD

The Life of Shabkar

I DECIDED TO TRANSLATE THE LIFE OF SHABKAR, WHICH IS NEARLY A THOUSAND pages, because I found it to be one of the most inspiring biographies of spiritual literature and felt sorry at the idea that it could only be read by those who can read Tibetan. His life story makes one wish that the duration of one's spiritual practice may be that of one's life.

Shabkar was born in 1781 among the Nyingmapa yogins of the Rekong region in Amdo, the remote northeast province of Greater Tibet. These yogins were renowned for their mastery of the secret Mantrayana practices and gathered in the thousands to engage in meditations and rituals. They were much admired, and sometimes feared, for their magical powers. The yogins of Rekong were also famous for their long hair, often 6 feet long, which they wore coiled on the top of their heads.

From a very early age, Shabkar showed a strong inclination toward the contemplative life. Even his childhood games were related to the teachings of Lord Buddha. By the age of six or seven, he had already developed a desire to practice. Visions, similar to those experienced in advanced *dzogchen* practice, came to him naturally.

Despite his deep affection for his mother and respect for his family, Shabkar managed to resist their repeated requests that he marry. He eventually left home to pursue wholeheartedly his spiritual aims. Totally determined to renounce worldly concerns, Shabkar received full monastic ordination at the age of twenty and entered a meditation retreat. He let his hair grow long again, as was customary for retreatants who did not waste time in nonessential activities. As a sign of having accomplished certain yogic practices, he wore a white shawl rather than the traditional red shawl, although he continued to wear the patched lower robe characteristic of a fully ordained monk. This rather unconventional attire occasionally attracted sarcastic comments from strangers, to whom Shabkar would reply with humorous songs.

Shabkar left his native land behind and traveled south of Rekong to meet his main teacher, the Dharma King Ngakyi Wangpo (1736–1807). After receiving complete instructions from the Dharma King, Shabkar practiced for five years in the wilderness of Tseshung, where his meditation experiences and realization flourished. He then meditated for three years on a small island, Tsonying, the "Heart of the Lake," in the Kokonor, the Blue Lake of Amdo. He became renowned as Shabkar Lama, the "White Footprint Lama," because he spent years in meditation at Mount Kailash, below Milarepa's Cave of Miracles, near the famous White Footprint, one of the four footprints said to have been left by Buddha Shakyamuni when he traveled miraculously to Kailash. It is also said that Shabkar was called "White Foot" because wherever he would set his feet, the land would become "white," meaning that through his teachings the minds of the people would be turned toward the holy Dharma.

In Shabkar's hagiography and songs, we receive a privileged and intimate view of the world of the Buddhist practitioner, a world of intense self-discipline, but also of humor, vision, and joy. Like Milarepa, of whom he was said to be an incarnation, Shabkar expressed his teachings, advice, and accounts of spiritual experiences in the form of songs. In his native province of Amdo, excerpts of his life and songs were often read to the dying, instead of the *Bardo Thodrol,* the so-called *Tibetan Book of the Dead.*

In a simple yet elegant form, Shabkar describes all the steps of his spiritual path, culminating in the teachings of the Great Perfection, *dzogchen.* He tells how, having become disillusioned with worldly activities, he sought a spiritual master, developed confidence in him, and followed his instructions. By practicing with complete dedication, in the end he himself became an enlightened master capable of contributing immensely to the welfare of beings. Shabkar's account of his progress along the spiritual path is so straightforward, heartfelt, and unaffected that one is encouraged to believe that similar deep faith and diligence would allow anyone else to achieve the same result.

135

Shabkar's didactic songs teach us the value and significance of human life, the meaning of death and impermanence, the law of *karma,* and the inherent suffering of *samsara.* He often extols the benefits of renunciation, the need to rely on a qualified teacher and to cultivate devotion, the view of emptiness imbued with the heart of great compassion, and finally, the realization of the Great Perfection—the primordial, unchanging purity of all phenomena, the innate Buddha-nature. Not only does Shabkar explain all this, he urges and inspires us to make these teachings a living experience, a part of ourselves.

Shabkar was always attentive to protecting animals in danger. He gave up eating meat after seeing sheep and goats slaughtered in Lhasa.[1] Feeling unbearable compassion for all animals in the world who are killed for food, he went before the Jowo Rinpoche, the famed Crowned Buddha statue of Lhasa, prostrated himself there, and made this vow: "From today on, I give up the negative act of eating the flesh of beings, each one whom was once my parent." He would also ransom the lives of animals going to be slaughtered, and set them free. At Tsonying Island, he used to sit by the shore of the lake during the summer to protect the baby birds who couldn't yet fly from birds of prey. The fledglings soon understood that he was protecting them and would gather near him whenever an eagle approached.

Shabkar's search for sacred places took him to many other solitary retreats, to the arduous pilgrimage of the Ravines of Tsari, to Mount Kailash, and to the Lapchi Snow Range. He spent many years in the very caves where Milarepa and other saints had lived and meditated. Wandering as a homeless yogin, teaching all beings, from bandits to wild animals, Shabkar's pilgrimages brought him as far as Nepal, where, in the

Kathmandu Valley, he had the entire spire of the Bodhnath Stupa covered with the gold his devotees had offered him.

In 1828, at the age of forty-seven, Shabkar returned to Amdo, where he tirelessly helped others through his extraordinary compassion. He spent the last twenty years of his life teaching disciples, promoting peace in the area, and practicing meditation in retreat at various sacred places, primarily at his hermitage at Tashikhyil. The reputation of Shabkar, the perfect hermit, spread far and wide, inspiring another great renunciate, Patrul Rinpoche,[2] to travel from Kham to Amdo to meet him. Unfortunately, after Patrul had gone only halfway he heard that Shabkar had passed away, whereupon he prostrated a hundred times in the direction of Amdo and sang a supplication for Shabkar's swift rebirth. He then added, "Compassion and love are the root of Dharma. I think that there was no one more compassionate than Shabkar in this world. I had nothing special to ask, no teachings to request from him, no teaching to offer him; I simply wanted to gather some merit by seeing his face."

Shabkar died in 1851. His life story can move one to tears or to laughter; but above all, as Kyabje Dilgo Khyentse Rinpoche[3] said, "As one reads it, one's mind cannot resist being turned toward the Dharma."

[1] His powerful admonition against eating meat is one of Shabkar's favorite themes.

[2] Patrul Rinpoche, Orgyen Jigme Chekyi Wangpo (1808–1887), was also known as Dzogchen Palge Tulku. Uncompromising in his interpretation of the teachings, Patrul Rinpoche lived as he taught, wandering all over eastern Tibet, taking shelter in mountain caves or under forest trees, free of all the trappings of wealth, position, and self-importance.

[3] Kyabje Dilgo Khyentse Rinpoche (1910–1991) was one of the greatest Nyingma masters of our times, and the most exemplary present-day exponent of the nonsectarian movement.

Matthieu Ricard, a former biology researcher, is a writer and photojournalist who has been a Buddhist monk for over twenty years. He is an interpreter for the Dalai Lama and served as Khyentse Rinpoche's assistant for the last fourteen years of Rinpoche's life. Ricard has translated numerous works about Buddhism.

If I had known I could get there with yoga,
I wouldn't be dying right now.

FRANK

CHERI CLAMPETT

A Knowing Beyond Words

ALTHOUGH I AM PASSIONATE ABOUT THE MANY WAYS IN WHICH YOGA CAN positively affect the quality of people's lives, my focus as a certified yoga therapist and instructor has always been on its healing aspects. To this end, I have spent much of the last ten years teaching yoga to people living with cancer, AIDS, and other ailments. Yoga has tremendous physical benefits, toning the internal organs, increasing strength and flexibility, improving circulation, and reducing stress levels. Even more important, yoga empowers individuals to take an active role in their healing process. Yoga's ancient techniques guide them into deeper states of consciousness, an ideal complement to traditional healing treatments.

During the summer of 1994, I held a free weekly yoga class at the Carl Bean AIDS Care Center, a hospice in East Los Angeles. I was used to offering yoga to people who were ill; many of my students had died, and yet I had never worked specifically with people who were in the process of dying. Although my focus may have been on yoga's healing aspects, the healing path for someone about to die looks very different. This class proved to be a powerful catalyst for my own growth and learning. It also provided me with one of my most poignant yoga memories.

Frank was a favorite student of mine who came each week to the hospice class. Like many of the people in this specific hospice, he had acquired the AIDS virus through IV drug use. Frank showed an enthusiasm for yoga, and would often ask me questions after class. His health seemed to be improving, and he was even talking about going home to be with his family. After each class I would invite everyone to come to a seated position for meditation. Those who weren't comfortable sitting would stay

lying down. After a few minutes of quiet and our closing salute, *namaste*, we would take time to share our experiences. On that day, I noticed Frank looked different. His eyes were bright and he seemed quite moved. When it came time for him to share, he said, "My whole life I have been trying to find this feeling. I felt totally peaceful, like I was floating. I imagine this is what death is going to feel like. For years I used drugs to feel good, to have this same feeling. If I had known I could get there with yoga, I wouldn't be dying right now."

This moment touched me deeply because it reminded me of my first experience with yoga, one that changed the course of my life. In my mid-twenties, I found myself in a yoga class at a new studio near my house. I had always been curious about this ancient practice but was afraid to explore it beyond imagining the wild postures I had seen in photographs. With the help of two good friends, I bypassed my fear and there I was, listening to the teacher guide us through a series of completely foreign physical postures. I found everything extremely difficult and was impressed by the challenge, realizing that many of my concepts of yoga were inaccurate. When we moved into the last position, lying flat on our backs in *Savasana*, also called the corpse pose, for final relaxation, I felt pleased. Now this was a posture I could do! What followed was an experience I'll never forget. After finding that position of comfort guided by the teacher, I began to move into a place that was unfamiliar to me. I felt heavy and relaxed but not sleepy. I began to feel my body in a way that was new to me. It was like listening to an old friend that I cared about. The communication was a whisper of sensation and a knowing beyond words. I felt a tremendous sadness flow through me. I realized that for as long as I could remember I had not been listening to my body, and there was so much it needed me to hear. Tears streamed down my face as I allowed myself to feel it all. At that moment, I became aware that something was wrong with my body.

For several months I had been experiencing a sharp, deep, shooting pain. I usually brushed it off because it didn't last. Even though the pain was severe when it happened, I would rationalize it as caused by something I had eaten or any number of other possibilities. But as I listened to that place in my body where the pain was, a warning came that was so strong that I knew it was time for me to pay attention. I went to see my doctor shortly afterward. After a maze of tests, I discovered that my body indeed needed me to listen. The signals it had been giving me were due to the cancer it was fighting. Immediately following my diagnosis I was rushed in for surgery. Fortunately, the cancer was caught early and I was spared further treatment. That experience made me want to teach yoga and share with others what had given me so much, perhaps even saved my life.

In the years since this experience, my journey with yoga has given me a tremendous respect for the power of any spiritual practice that leads the focus inside. As a teacher of yoga I strive to create a safe space for my students to journey there and feel the deeper parts of their being, which is where the greatest insights and transformations occur. My first experience of yoga and Frank's experience feeling peace illustrate how, in one moment of inner listening, a life can be deeply touched and forever changed in a positive way.

Cheri Clampett is a respected yoga teacher. For the last ten years, her teaching has focused on people with cancer, AIDS, or physical injuries. Currently, Clampett leads Therapeutic Yoga Training, an innovative course she created to show nurses, physical therapists, and other yoga teachers how to apply yoga to patient care. Her spiritual practice includes yoga, meditation, and the belief that love is the ultimate healer.

The real miracle is not to walk on water, but to walk on the earth,
to be alive in the present moment.

THICH NHAT HANH

THICH NHAT HANH

The Peace of the Divine Reality

I WOULD LIKE TO SHARE A POEM WITH YOU, WRITTEN BY A FRIEND WHO DIED AT the age of twenty-eight in Saigon, about thirty years ago. After he died, people found many beautiful poems he had written, and I was startled when I read this poem:

> *Standing quietly by the fence,*
> *you smile your wondrous smile.*
> *I am speechless, and my senses are filled*
> *by the sounds of your beautiful song.*
> *Beginningless and endless.*
> *I bow deeply to you.*

"You" refers to a flower, a dahlia. That morning as he passed by a fence, he saw that little flower very deeply, and struck by the sight of it, he stopped and wrote that poem.

I enjoy this poem very much. You may think that the poet was a Zen master because his way of looking and seeing things is very deep. But he was just an ordinary person, a poet. I don't exactly know how or why he was able to see like that, but it is exactly the way we practice Buddhist meditation, the practice of mindfulness. We try to be in touch with life in the present moment and look deeply into the things that happen to us in the present moment. We do that while we drink tea, while we talk, while we sit down, and so on. The secret of success is that you are yourself, you are really yourself, and when you are really yourself, you can encounter life in the present moment.

During the Last Supper, Jesus Christ told his disciples, "This piece of bread is my flesh. Eat it." That was a radical statement. He must have noticed that his twelve friends were not awake, and when he saw that, he wanted to say something strong to wake them up, to help them live fully in the present moment. He also told them, "This wine is my blood. Drink it." Eating bread and really eating the bread, drinking wine and really drinking the wine, looking at a flower, looking at the eyes of a child, at the Kingdom of God, at the Pure Land, is right here.

There is another story about a flower, a story well known in Zen circles. One day the Buddha held up a flower in front of an audience of 1,250 monks. He did not say anything for quite a long time. Suddenly, he smiled. He smiled because someone in the audience smiled at him and at the flower. The name of that monk was Mahakashyapa. That story has been discussed by many generations of Buddhists, and people continue to look for its meaning. To me, the meaning is quite simple. When someone holds up a flower and shows it to you, he wants you to see it. And if you keep thinking, you miss the flower. The person who was not thinking, who was just himself, was able to encounter the flower in depth, and he smiled.

That is the problem of life. If we are not here, if we are not in the present moment, fully ourselves, we miss everything. When a child presents himself to you, with his smile, and if you are not really there, you are thinking about the future or you are thinking about the past, or you are preoccupied by other problems, then the child is not really there for you. The technique of being alive, of living in the divine and earthly realities simultaneously, is to go back to yourself. Then the child will appear like a marvelous reality; then you can see her smile and embrace her.

Living in this marvelous reality, living in peace, is something we all want. But I would like to ask: Do we have the capacity of enjoying peace? If peace is there, will we be able to enjoy it, or will we find it boring? To me, peace and happiness and joy and life go together, and we can experience the peace of the divine reality right in the present moment. It is available, inside us and around us. If we are not able to enjoy that peace, how can we make peace grow?

When I have a toothache, I discover that not having a toothache is a wonderful thing. That is peace. I had to have a toothache to be enlightened, to know that not having one is wonderful. My nontoothache is peace, is joy. But when I do not have a toothache, I do not seem to be very happy. Therefore, to look deeply at the present moment and see that I have a non-toothache, that can make me very happy already.

147

I know a doctor who lost her eyesight because during the night, she used the wrong eye drops, and a few months later, she was not able to see anything. Every time she wants to remember the lines on her son's face, she has to call him close to her and rediscover those lines with her fingertips. To her, to be able to see things would be a miracle. She says that she would be in paradise if she could recover her eyesight. According to that criterion, most of us are already in paradise, because we have eyes capable of seeing. If we open our eyes we can see the blue sky, the white clouds, the clear stream, the flowers, the beautiful child. We need only to be mindful that we have eyes, and they can make us very happy. An element of peace is already here.

There are so many things that can provide us with peace. Next time you take a shower or bath, I suggest you hold your big toes in mindfulness. We pay attention to everything except our toes. When we hold our toes in mindfulness and smile at them, we will find that our bodies have been very kind to us. We know that any cell in our toes can turn cancerous, but our toes have been behaving very well, avoiding that kind of problem. Yet, we have not been nice to them at all. These kinds of practices can bring us happiness.

When we contemplate the body in the body, we can discover these kinds of things. When we contemplate the feelings in the feelings, we discover there are many beautiful seeds of feelings in us. We can help ourselves to happiness and joy because if we do not, we shall be in touch only with the painful aspects of life. We usually ask "What is wrong?" and focus all our energy and attention on that while our happiness grows thinner and thinner. We neglect what is right, what is wonderful in us and around us. The practice of mindfulness of what is *not* wrong is wonderful.

We were able to smile a lot when we were young, but life is so hard that when we grow up, we hardly smile. I know people who have not smiled for ten or twenty years. The seeds of the smiles in the depths of their consciousnesses have not had a chance to arise for a long time. They only ask, "What is wrong?" So, asking the questions "What is right? What is not wrong?" is a good beginning. By asking in this way and paying attention to these fresh elements that are healing and refreshing, we are able to heal ourselves, to grow, and to generate joy and happiness for our sakes and for the sake of people who live around us.

The Buddha delivered a sermon on the mindfulness of breathing. He proposed sixteen exercises for us to practice. These exercises are wonderful. The first exercise is so simple: "Breathing in, I know that I am breathing in. Breathing out, I know that I am breathing out." Just that. If you find these sentences too long, you can say just two words: "in, out." You breathe in and you know it is an in-breath, and you breathe out and say "out," recognizing it as an out-breath. That is all.

I think Mahakashyapa was practicing this mindfulness when the Buddha held up the flower, and that is why the encounter between him and the flower was possible. All the others were thinking, and their thinking blocked the encounter. Thinking is important, but most of our thinking is useless. It seems that we have cassette tapes in our heads, always running, day and night. We think of this and we think of that, and it is difficult for us to stop. With a cassette, we can just press the Stop button. But with our thinking, we do not have such a button. So when we think too much, we worry, we cannot sleep, we block our encounters with the present moment.

According to this method of breathing, when we breathe in and out, we stop thinking, because "in, out" are not thoughts—they are only words that help us concentrate on our breathing. If we keep breathing in and out and smiling for a few minutes, we become quite refreshed. We recover ourselves, and then we can encounter the flower, the piece of bread, the wine, the child. We do not miss anything that is happening in the present moment.

Breathing in and out is very important, and it is enjoyable! You know, when you have a stuffed nose, you cannot enjoy breathing. When you have asthma, you cannot enjoy breathing. But when the air is clean and when you do not have asthma, it is wonderful to breathe. To me, breathing is a joy that I cannot miss. Every day I practice breathing, and in my small meditation room is this sentence: "Breathe, you are alive!" Just breathing and smiling can make us very happy, and when we breathe consciously we recover ourselves completely and encounter life in the present moment. To me, this is the Kingdom of Heaven. The real miracle is not to walk on water, but to walk on the earth, to be alive in the present moment. If we live in mindfulness, it is possible to encounter God right in the present moment while we are washing the dishes, looking at a flower, looking in the eyes of a child.

When we are in touch with the refreshing, peaceful, and healing elements within ourselves and around us, we learn how to cherish and protect these things and to make them grow. These are the elements of peace and happiness available to us anytime. If we do not look closely at these simple things, we may find them boring.

There are people who cannot enjoy simple pleasures, and that is why they seek drugs, alcohol, sexual misconduct, and many other things that destroy them, their bodies, their minds, and their families, and cause their children and grandchildren to suffer. If we educate ourselves and our children on how to enjoy peace in the present moment and to be happy with the refreshing and healing elements that are available, we will avoid these kinds of traps. Life can be found only in the present moment. The past is gone, the future is not yet here, and if we do not go back to ourselves in the present moment, we cannot be in touch with life.

Thich Nhat Hanh is a Buddhist monk, poet, peace activist, and the author of *Being Peace, The Miracle of Mindfulness,* and many other books. He lives in a monastic community in southwestern France called Plum Village, where he teaches, writes, gardens, and works to help refugees worldwide. He conducts retreats throughout the world on the art of mindful living.

I see two birds on the same branch.
One eats the sweet fruit, the other looks on sadly.
The first bird wonders, "In what prison does he live?"
The second marvels, "How can he rejoice?"

RAMAYANA

BO LOZOFF

The Samurai and the Zen Master

I FIRST HEARD THE STORY OF THE SAMURAI AND THE ZEN MASTER FROM RAM DASS in the early 1970s. A young Samurai warrior stood respectfully before an aged Zen master and said, "Master, teach me about Heaven and Hell." The master snapped his head up in disgust and said, "Teach you about Heaven and Hell? Why, I doubt that you could even learn to keep your own sword from rusting! You ignorant fool! How dare you suppose that you could understand anything I might have to say! I am a great master and you are nothing but a wretch!" The old man went on and on, becoming even more insulting, while the young swordsman's surprise turned first to confusion and then to hot anger, rising by the moment. Master or no master, who can insult a Samurai and live? At last, with teeth clenched and blood boiling in fury, the warrior drew his sword and prepared to end the old man's sharp tongue and life in one furious stroke. At that very moment, the master looked straight into his eyes and said gently, "That's Hell."

Even at the peak of his rage, the Samurai realized that the master had indeed given him the teaching he had asked for. He had hounded him into a living hell, driven by his uncontrolled anger and pride. The young warrior, now deeply humbled, sheathed his sword and bowed low to this great and courageous spiritual teacher. Looking up into the master's smiling face, he felt more love and compassion than he had ever felt in all his life.

At that point the master raised his index finger and said kindly, "And that's Heaven."

Recognizing the power of our own minds to drive us into the realms of hell or the realms of heaven is invaluable for those of us who work or live in brutal environments such as prisons. We have a sacred duty to strive toward the eradication of injustice, poverty, racism, and all other forms of oppression and degradation. But those conditions are not emotional states, they do not guarantee heaven or hell in and of themselves. I know prisoners in some of the most horrendous, unfair environments imaginable who live closer to heaven than many affluent or middle-class people. And we have all seen examples of the most privileged people on earth whose lives seem like hell. This principle has helped me to take personal responsibility for my states of mind and to encourage my readers and listeners to do the same.

In two of my books, *Deep & Simple* and *It's a Meaningful Life,* I have included a vow practice that goes something like this: "I vow to refrain from blaming others for my negative states of mind. I vow to refrain from blaming circumstances for my negative states of mind." People in Kindness House, the spiritual community where I live, work frequently with this vow. If we get sick, have a lousy night's sleep, or receive terrible news, we resist making the assumption that any such circumstances justify irritability or other forms of negativity. It's a very useful practice in seeing the unnecessary psychological programming we tend to follow blindly.

Bo Lozoff and his wife, Sita, are directors of the Human Kindness Foundation in Durham, North Carolina. They have worked with prisoners for over twenty-five years. Lozoff's first book, *We're All Doing Time,* has been translated into several languages. His other books include *Lineage and Other Stories, Just Another Spiritual Book, Deep & Simple: A Spiritual Path for Modern Times,* and *It's a Meaningful Life: It Just Takes Practice.* In 1994, Lozoff and Sita received the Temple Award for Creative Altruism. In 1999, Lozoff was awarded an honorary doctorate from the Chicago Theological Seminary.

I sit at the table of unknowing and invite you to join me there.

❖

JACQUIE BELLON

You're Preapproved: Accept Today

I DON'T KNOW WHO I AM, OR WHO MY MOTHER IS, OR WHY SHE GAVE ME AWAY AT three months, just when I was beginning to smile. I was born in Vietnam, left it at age six and lived in the south of France with my grandmother until the age of twelve when I joined my parents in Hollywood, where they had established themselves. At age seventeen I was told that my biological mother was Vietnamese, my biological father was French, that they had died in the war; and that I had been adopted with great love, given every opportunity for a life full of possibilities and choices, and I should be grateful. I don't look particularly Vietnamese. I can look Mexican, American Indian, South American. I look "Third World" and can pass unnoticed in countries where people are small and dark. But I grew up thinking I was white. I felt guilty for wanting to know more about my history, but little by little, in fits and starts, fragments were reluctantly offered.

When my son was born, my adoptive mother told me another story. After my biological father died, his brother felt responsible for my care. He took me from my birth mother and placed me with my adoptive parents, who were his friends. My birth mother came to reclaim me, and when my adoptive mother complained to my uncle, he supposedly said, "I'll take care of it," and brought me back to her once again. "Your mother sold you," I was told. Eventually she married, bore several children, and lived in Hanoi. I no longer knew what was true or what time and individual perceptions had distorted and realized that no one else knew either. We had all made up stories to fit our belief systems. However, my birth certificate surfaced and on it my Vietnamese name, Do Thi Ba. My son was born with a Mongolian spot on his buttocks, so I knew that the Vietnamese part was true. By this time, America was involved in a full-blown war in Vietnam and I was an American citizen. I was both sides, torn and conflicted, at war with myself.

I tried for years to find answers and to categorize everything into neat packages, labeled and tucked away in boxes on shelves and in file cabinets. I tried to go back to past lives and cellular memories, endured deep tissue bodywork, undertook years of weepy therapy, rummaging through composted, distorted memories under the guidance of various well-meaning people. I raised a child, explored Zen meditation and yoga, and joined a gym. I became a white-water guide, began to downhill ski after age forty, kept a journal and illustrated it. I doggedly pursued a career as an artist, held a multitude of freelance jobs to keep afloat, and traveled the world on a shoestring. On an island in Thailand, sitting on a hot, sandy beach, staring at the horizon line, I came to the realization that transformation could manifest in any number of ways and that I had not reached some higher realm. Instead I had become a vegetable, a sea cucumber, or limp lettuce. I went back to Vietnam to find my mother and parts of myself.

I traveled halfway across the globe on a pilgrimage of sorts, hungry for revelations and insights, for a deep understanding. I arrived instead at a place of exhaustion and emptiness that felt more like bankruptcy. My mother died without ever telling me any more pieces of the story, wounded because she felt rejected. My father survived her by five years, plunging into a deep depression and atrophying in body and spirit, until finally he was unable to speak at all. The day I was called to his side my husband moved out to be with his lover. I sat with my father, breathing with him until he stopped, imagining that his last undecipherable mumblings were some of the details I needed to know. With their deaths, the possibility of a fuller picture of myself became dimmer. It would be a few more years of yearning and searching until I was sufficiently humbled into joyful surrender.

One day I came to rest on a wooden chair at a round table in a house I had built, on land I had cleared of brush by hand with someone I had loved. I finally realized that I didn't know, would never know, and that it was okay. I could sit at the table of unknowing and have a glass of wine. I didn't need all the facts. I could rejoice in the mystery of living. The questions are numberless and the openings limitless. I was meant to live with an open mind and heart; I was free to enjoy life as it is. Even the unsolicited mail from credit-card companies could teach me something when it assured me, "You're preapproved, accept today!"

159

Jacqueline Bellon first became interested in Zen when she was in her early twenties and studied with Sasaki Roshi in Los Angeles. Her next teacher, many years later, was Joko Beck. Bellon, a painter and writer, lives in the Sierra Nevada foothills of California.

As Yunyan was sweeping the ground, Daowu said, "Too busy."
Yunyan said, "You should know there's one who isn't busy."
Daowu said, "If so, then there's a second moon."
Yunyan held up the broom and said, "Which moon is this?"

A ZEN *KOAN*

SUSAN MOON

Who Isn't Busy?

As much as I love it, my job editing *Turning Wheel*[1] is a constant source of stress; no sooner do I meet one deadline than the next one rolls in. I'm a writer and a writing teacher, a parent, an aunt, a sister. I take photography and yoga classes; I belong to a Dharma study group, a writing group, and a Zen seminar. Periodically I resolve to simplify my life, but as soon as I resign from one committee, a new project pops up that I can't resist. In the midst of this whirlwind, I long for inner peace.

Over twenty-five years ago, I went to Tassajara Zen Mountain Monastery (in the coastal mountains of California) as a visitor during the summer guest season. The monks struck a chord in me, slapping along the gravel paths in their sandals and black robes, bowing to each other, carrying tea, or sweeping. It was there I had my first *zazen* instruction, and when I returned home to Berkeley, I joined the Berkeley Zen Center, where I've been practicing ever since.

The dream of returning to slap my own way down those paths in my own black robes stayed with me. Several years ago, after my children had flown the coop, I arranged to take off from my normal working life to go to Tassajara for a formal three-month winter practice period. I found other people to take care of the job, the house, the car, the mail, and the cactus plant in my absence. I had to have robes made for myself—an under robe and an outer robe. I chose the fabric, found the seamstress, and went for fittings. I borrowed various other things to complete my monk costume: a special kind of blouse called a *jubon,* a special kind of rope belt, and a sitting bench in case I needed a break from my *zafu* (cushion). I had to get long underwear, a flashlight, a hot-water bottle, a thermos, and waterproof clogs.

164

I was excited and nervous on the January day when I finally left my Berkeley life behind and entered the still mountains. It was snowing as the Tassajara van carried another entering monk and me over the pass on the long dirt road, and when we came down into the deep fold in the mountains where the monastery lies, a light wet snow still stuck to the ground. I had crossed the threshold! Here in this sacred place, surely I would find peace within my heart!

Dark winter morning after dark winter morning, day after day, sleepy evening after sleepy evening, I sat in the *zendo* in my black monk's robes. My belt was carefully tied in the prescribed manner, with a slipknot at either side of my waist. I followed the schedule with devotion, never missing a period of *zazen* and never coming late.

And here, sitting still at last in the mountains, my mind jumped like a flea. It was as bad as ever. Even here, where I didn't have to worry about meetings or deadlines or returning phone calls or e-mail messages or getting the oil in the car changed, my mind raced wildly through the emptiness, looking for something to do. I considered the question of whether to wash my long underwear today or tomorrow. I told myself to follow my breathing, and found myself calculating how many breaths I breathed in a period of *zazen,* how many periods of *zazen* there were in the practice period, how many breaths I would breathe during my time as a monk. I planned my diet: I'd allow myself seconds in the third bowl but not in the middle two. I went around the *zendo* in my mind guessing the ages of my fellow monks—how many people were older and how many were younger than I was? What was the average age?

I'd catch myself and try to come back to the present moment. What the hell did I think I was doing? Why was I here? Why was I torturing myself? I felt like a hypocrite. My mind was like a dog that needed a bone to chew on, but there was no bone, and so my mind gnawed on itself. I was certain that there was something terribly wrong with me. Everybody else knew how to meditate. Everybody was getting enlightened but me. The others looked so peaceful I was sure they couldn't be wasting their precious human birth as I was. I hated myself. The busyness inside my head was as noisy and as devoid of meaning as the busyness in the outside world. I was wearing my robes and sitting on my cushion, but I wasn't liberated.

One afternoon I sat on a bench in the garden during a break, under apple blossoms, in the sun. I was grateful to be out of the *zendo*. I thought of the *koan* in which one monk asks the other, "What is the most difficult thing?" And the second monk answers, "To wear these robes and not understand the Great Matter." That was just how I felt. It was agony to struggle and struggle and still *not* understand, not know who I was or why I was there. I felt that I was failing, over and over, moment by moment.

I spoke to Reb Anderson, the teacher leading the practice period, about the relentless busyness of my mind. I told him I was being driven mad by the chaos of my thoughts, the plans, the dreams, the fantasies, the obsessions. I wanted to find something simple and true inside myself. And I was angry with myself for having bad *zazen*.

Reb said, "Read Case 21 of the *Book of Serenity*. Memorize it; study it." I got the book out of the Tassajara library and read the case hungrily.

> As Yunyan was sweeping the ground, Daowu said, "Too busy."
> Yunyan said, "You should know there's one who isn't busy."
> Daowu said, "If so, then there's a second moon."
> Yunyan held up the broom and said, "Which moon is this?"

What a wonderful gift this *koan* was! I felt as if it had been written especially for me—after all, not only was I busy, but my name was Moon. And here, at last, was some comfort. Even in the midst of Yunyan's sweeping, there was a Yunyan who wasn't busy.

Daowu challenged him: "If so, then there's a second moon." I take that to mean, "I see a Yunyan who's sweeping, and you're telling me there's a Yunyan who isn't busy. You're telling me there are two Yunyans? You might as well be saying there are two moons."

And Yunyan's answer brings the two together: he holds up the broom. In the moment of his question—"Which moon is this?"—I see the broom hanging there, still, in the air. It's not sweeping, but it's the tool of sweeping. Is the broom busy? It's both busy and not busy. It's Yunyan being both busy and not busy.

Reb pointed me to this *koan* to help me with *zazen*. He wanted me to understand that no matter how busy my mind was during *zazen*, there was always some part of me who was not busy, who was just sitting there, upright, facing the wall. And I was greatly reassured. I realized that I couldn't get away from the one who was not busy even if I tried. Sometimes I imagine my spinal column as the one who isn't busy, upright in the middle of my body, while the thoughts swirl, the heart beats, the blood rushes around, the air goes in and out.

During that practice period, I didn't exactly discover the meaning of life, but I stopped making war on myself during *zazen;* and when I left Tassajara to return to the world, I took Yunyan and Daowu with me.

As time went by, the *koan* helped me in other contexts. I appreciated it at the most literal level. Yunyan was busy sweeping the ground. In the sometimes overwhelming busyness of daily life there's always one who's not busy. As Thich Nhat Hanh reminds us, washing dishes is a kind of *zazen,* too.

I've learned that sometimes it's not enough for me just to have faith that the one who's not busy is there somewhere inside the tornado. Periodically I need to coax her out of her shell, even if just for a few minutes to remind myself she's really there. Sometimes, in the middle of the day at the Buddhist Peace Fellowship office, we turn off the phones, faxes, computers, and buzzing fluorescent lights, and sit for ten minutes in silence. Sometimes, on my way home from the office, I stop at the Berkeley Zen Center for evening *zazen*. Sometimes I just turn off the car radio and drive across town in silence, thinking of nothing in particular. Sometimes I lie down for five minutes on the sofa with an eye pillow on my face. You can think of these activities as forms of stress reduction, or practice, but now I also think of them as getting in touch with the one who is not busy, so that when I *am* busy, I have more confidence that the one who is *not* is there as well.

When a wheel turns, the circumference moves the fastest. As you go toward the center, the motion is slower and slower. At the very center of the circle is a point that is completely still. That's where Buddha sits.

Yunyan and Daowu have also helped me think about the relationship between activism and meditation. "Yunyan was sweeping the ground." How can you sweep the ground? There's no end to it. It's like saying, "Yunyan was working to bring peace to the world. Yunyan was trying to save all sentient beings." Daowu said, "Too busy." He might have meant, "You've taken on too much, little brother. More leaves will fall as soon as you've swept these up."

I was an activist before I was a Buddhist, and when I started sitting, I used to worry that every moment on my cushion was stolen from saving the world. I don't feel that now. I know that without a spiritual practice, my actions in pursuit of social justice would become bankrupt, and I would burn out. I also know that for me, a spiritual life without any application to social concerns would lose its power. But everybody has a different balance. I want to live in a world that has room for monasteries, where people can spend a lifetime in meditation. I feel they are doing it for me.

A few years ago, after my practice period at Tassajara, I went to a conference in Cambodia. There I met Maha Ghosananda, senior monk of Cambodia, now in his eighties. I stayed in his temple in Phnom Penh, and spent a fair amount of time in his presence. I even had the opportunity to interview him for *Turning Wheel,* though he's practically impossible to interview: he's a man of few words and many smiles. He travels all over the world, going to peace conferences and summit meetings, trying to bring the suffering in Cambodia to the international eye and working against land mines and war. In spite of being a very busy man, he always seems calm and peaceful. Every year for the last seven or eight years he's led a peace walk through Cambodia, asking for reconciliation, and risking injury from land mines or civil war. One year, two peace walkers were killed, a Cambodian monk and nun, when they were caught in the crossfire between government forces and the Khmer Rouge. But the following year, Maha Ghosananda and hundreds of others walked again for peace.

In the early 1980s, when there were big demonstrations at the Livermore Nuclear Weapons Laboratory, I was one of hundreds of people who sat in the road obstructing traffic. I remember how quiet it was in that moment of sitting down and holding hands. Workers in their cars honked to get by, a phalanx of California Highway Patrol officers dressed in full riot gear marched down on us, and our friends and supporters called out to us, singing, and cheering us on. In the midst of all that excitement and fear, the one who was not busy just sat there, upright, until she was handcuffed and led away.

There are as many ways to save beings as there are beings. I don't think everybody has to be an activist in the obvious sense. (I haven't been doing much demonstrating myself lately.) But I do believe that everybody needs to find a broom.

The *koan* tells me that sometimes I'm a full moon and sometimes I'm a crescent moon, but I'm just one moon. The *koan* reminds me that I can be both the broom that sweeps the ground and the broom that's held up. I can be both the elder brother, quick on the draw, ready with a testing question, and the younger brother, steady, persevering, willing to not understand for years and years. I can be busy with many activities and have peace in my heart at the same time.

When Reb told me to study this *koan,* I memorized it right away, and regularly repeated it to myself. One morning during work period, soon after Case 21 had become a kind of mantra for me, I was sweeping leaves off a little wooden bridge. Reb happened to come along the path and I held up the broom and waved it at him. "Which moon is this?"

---

[1] *Turning Wheel* is the journal of the Buddhist Peace Fellowship.

Susan Moon is the author of a book of fiction, *The Life and Letters of Tofu Roshi,* and coeditor, with Lenore Friedman, of the anthology *Being Bodies: Buddhist Women on the Paradox of Embodiment.* She is editor of *Turning Wheel,* the quarterly journal of the Buddhist Peace Fellowship. Her short stories and articles have appeared in many magazines and anthologies. Moon won a Pushcart Prize in 1992 and a National Endowment for the Arts grant for fiction in 1993. Moon joined the Berkeley Zen Center in 1976. She is the editor of a book of Reb Anderson's lectures, *Warm Smiles from Cold Mountains.* Moon is the mother of two grown sons and lives in Berkeley, California.

I'm always suspicious of the ones who say everything's going well. If you think that things are going well, then it's usually some kind of arrogance. If it's too easy for you, you just relax. You don't make a real effort, and therefore you never find out what it is to be fully human.

CHÖGYAM TRUNGPA RINPOCHE

PEMA CHÖDRÖN

Finding Our Own True Nature

IN ONE OF THE BUDDHA'S DISCOURSES, HE TALKS ABOUT THE FOUR KINDS OF horses: the excellent horse, the good horse, the poor horse, and the really bad horse. The excellent horse, according to the *sutra*,[1] moves before the whip even touches its back; just the shadow of the whip or the slightest sound from the driver is enough to make the horse move. The good horse runs at the lightest touch of the whip on its back. The poor horse doesn't go until it feels pain, and the very bad horse doesn't budge until the pain penetrates to the marrow of its bones.

When Shunryu Suzuki tells the story in his book *Zen Mind, Beginner's Mind,* he says that when people hear this *sutra,* they always want to be the best horse, but actually, when we sit, it doesn't matter whether we're the best horse or the worst horse. He goes on to say that, in fact, the really terrible horse is the best practitioner.

What I have realized through practicing is that practice isn't about being the best horse or the good horse or the poor horse or the worst horse. It's about finding our own true nature and speaking from that, acting from that. Whatever our quality is, that's our wealth and our beauty; that's what other people respond to.

Once I had an opportunity to talk with Chögyam Trungpa Rinpoche about the fact that I was not able to do my practice properly. I had just started the *Vajrayana*[3] practices and I was supposed to be visualizing. I couldn't visualize anything. I tried and tried but there was just nothing at all; I felt like a fraud doing the practice because it didn't feel natural to me. I was quite miserable because everybody else seemed to be having all kinds of visualizations and doing very well. He said, "I'm always suspicious of the ones who say everything's going well. If you think that things are going well, then it's usually some kind of arrogance. If it's too easy for you, you just relax. You don't make a real effort, and therefore you never find out what it is to be fully human." So he encouraged me by saying that as long as you have these kinds of doubts, your practice will be good. When you begin to think that everything is just perfect and feel complacent and superior to the others, watch out!

Dainin Katagiri Roshi once told a story about his own experience of being the worst horse. When he first came to the United States from Japan, he was a young monk in his late twenties. He had been a monk in Japan— where everything was so precise, so clean, so neat—for a long time. In the United States, his students were hippies with long, unwashed hair and ragged clothes and no shoes. He didn't like them. He couldn't help it—he just couldn't stand those hippies. Their style offended everything in him. He said, "So all I day I would give talks about compassion, and at night I would go home and weep and cry because I realized I had no compassion at all. Because I didn't like my students, therefore I had to work much harder to develop my heart." As Suzuki Roshi says in his talk, that's exactly the point: Because we find ourselves to be the worst horse, we are inspired to try harder.

At Gampo Abbey we had a Tibetan monk, Lama Sherap Tendar, teaching us to play the Tibetan musical instruments. We had forty-nine days in which to learn the music; we were also going to learn many other things, we thought, during that time. But as it turned out, for forty-nine days, twice a day, all we did was learn to play the cymbals and the drum and how they are played together. Every day we would practice and practice. We would practice on our own, and then we would play for Lama Sherap, who would sit there with this pained little look on his face. Then he would take our hands and show us how to play. Then we would do it by ourselves, and he would sigh. This went on for forty-nine days. He never said that we were doing well, but he was very sweet and very gentle. Finally, when it was all over and we had had our last performance, we were making toasts and remarks and Lama Sherap said, "Actually you were very good. You were very good right from the beginning, but I knew if I told you that you were good, you would stop trying." He was right. He had such a gentle way of encouraging us that it didn't make us angry with him and it didn't make us lose heart. It just made us feel that he knew the proper way to play the cymbals; he'd been playing these cymbals since he was a little boy, and we just had to keep trying. So for forty-nine days we really worked hard.

We can work with ourselves in the same way. We don't have to be harsh with ourselves when we think, sitting here, that our meditation or our *oryoki* or the way we are in the world is in the category of the worst horse. We could be very sympathetic with that and use it as a motivation to keep trying to develop ourselves, to find our own true nature. Not only will we find our own true nature, but we'll learn about other people because in our heart of hearts almost all of us feel that we are the worst horse. You might consider that you yourself are an arrogant person or you might consider that someone else is an arrogant person, but everybody who has ever felt even a moment of arrogance knows that arrogance is just a cover-up for really feeling that you're the worst horse and always trying to prove otherwise.

In his talk, Suzuki Roshi says that meditation and the whole process of finding your own true nature is one continuous mistake, and that rather than that being a reason for depression or discouragement, it's actually the motivation. When you find yourself slumping, that's the motivation to sit up, not out of self-denigration but actually out of pride in everything that occurs to you, pride in who you are just as you are, pride in the goodness or the fairness or the worstness of yourself—however you find yourself—some sort of sense of taking pride and using it to spur you on.

The Karma Kagyü lineage of Tibetan Buddhism, in which the students of Chögyam Trungpa are trained, is sometimes called the "mishap lineage," because of the ways in which the wise and venerated teachers of this lineage blew it time after time. First there was Tilopa, who was a madman, completely wild. His main student was Naropa. Naropa was so conceptual and intellectual that it took him twelve years of being "run over by a truck," of being put through all sorts of trials by his teacher, for him to begin to wake up. He was so conceptual that if somebody would tell him something, he would say, "Oh yes, but surely by *that* you must mean *this.*" He had that kind of mind. His main student was Marpa, who was famous for his intensely bad temper. He used to fly into rages, beat people, and yell at them. He was also a drunk. He was notorious for being incredibly stubborn. His student was Milarepa. Milarepa was a murderer! Rinpoche used to say that Marpa became a student of the Dharma because he thought he could make a lot of money by bringing texts back from India and translating them into Tibetan. His student Milarepa became a student because he was afraid he was going to go to hell for having murdered people—that scared him.

Milarepa's student was Gampopa (after whom Gampo Abbey is named). Because everything was easy for him, Gampopa was arrogant. For instance, the night before he met Gampopa for the first time, Milarepa said to some of his disciples, "Oh, someone who is destined to be my main student is going to come tomorrow. Whoever brings him to me will be greatly benefited." So when Gampopa arrived in the town, an old lady who saw him ran out and said, "Oh, Milarepa told us you were coming and that you were destined to be one of his main students, and I want my daughter to bring you to see him." So Gampopa, thinking, "I must be really hot stuff," went very proudly to meet Milarepa, sure that he would be greeted with great honor. However, Milarepa had had someone put him in a cave and wouldn't see Gampopa for three weeks.

As for Gampopa's main student, the first Karmapa, the only thing we know about him is that he was extremely ugly. He was said to look like a monkey. Also, there's one story about him and three other main disciples of Gampopa who were thrown out of the monastery for getting drunk and singing and dancing and breaking the monastic rules.

We could all take heart. These are the wise ones who sit in front of us, to whom we prostrate when we do prostrations. We can prostrate to them as an example of our own wisdom mind of enlightened beings, but perhaps it's also good to prostrate to them as confused, mixed-up people with a lot of neuroses, just like ourselves. They are good examples of people who never gave up on themselves and were not afraid of themselves, who therefore found their own genuine quality and their own true nature.

The point is that our true nature is not some ideal that we have to live up to. It's who we are right now, and that's what we can make friends with and celebrate.

[1] A discourse or teaching by the Buddha.
[2] The "diamond vehicle"; the practice of taking the result as the path.

Pema Chödrön is a fully ordained *bhikshuni* (Buddhist nun). She was the first American practitioner of the Vajrayana tradition to undergo full ordination. Born in 1936 in New York City, Chödrön has two grown children and one granddaughter. Formerly the director of Karma Dzong in Boulder, Colorado, Chödrön is now the director of Gampo Abbey, a monastic center in the Cape Breton Highlands of Nova Scotia, Canada. Pema Chödrön is the author of *When Things Fall Apart: Heart Advice for Difficult Times, Start Where You Are: A Guide to Compassionate Living,* and *The Wisdom of No Escape.*

The Tao described in words is not the real Tao.
Words cannot describe it.

TAO TE CHING

DALE PENDELL

Sauntering with Lao-tzu

THE BOOK CAME AS A GIFT, A DROP OF POISON THAT SLIPPED INTO MY THOUGHTS lightly, with unassuming metaphysics, and thus was able to evade the frontier defenses poised to attack any cosmic principle clothed in more theistic garb.

It was just a silly Peter Pauper Press book, and the translation, as I recognize now, not particularly scholarly. But it was compact and direct.

> *Man is subject to the laws of the earth,*
> *the earth is subject to the laws of the universe,*
> *the universe is subject to the laws of Tao, and*
> *Tao is subject to the laws of its own nature.*

The words evoked an image of flowing, light and vacuous, more like a subtle inclination emanating from "that which is" than as a thing itself.

> *Looked for, it cannot be seen.*

Thus it was all the more disturbing when I found that the accompanying philosophy was not only practical, including a theory of government and of history, but also radical:

> *the perfect state is small . . .*
> *they have weapons but no reason to show them . . .*

181

men forego writing, reckoning with knotted cord.
Do away with formal learning and you will not be annoyed by its
    multitude of details.

In my own wording,

182   *The scholar learns every day,*
the follower of the Way unlearns every day.

Lao-tzu had a way of turning things upside down. Over the years I collected many translations of the *Tao Te Ching,* but some verses remain in my memory in altered or hybrid form.

Red Pine translates verse 38:

when the Way is lost virtue appears
when virtue is lost kindness appears
when kindness is lost justice appears
when justice is lost ritual appears
ritual marks the waning of belief
and onset of confusion.

But in my memory the verse went more like

When the Way is lost there is custom,
when custom is lost, there is morality,
when morality is lost, there is ritual,
when ritual is lost, there are mere laws.

The gist is the same. Everywhere Lao-tzu challenges the entrenched ideas of "progress." The Old Ways of the Neolithic were still alive in Lao-tzu's century, though under assault from the centralizing forces of bronze and iron.

Lao-tzu taught leading from behind, that even better than leaders who were loved were leaders who were hardly noticed. He warned that fine-sounding words were not often true, and that when most people heard of the Tao, they just laughed.

Thus the truly wise want the unwanted and do not prize what is rare.
Study what is unstudied and preserve what is lost. Assist in the course of
nature but never interfere in it.

Lao-tzu offered the possibility of a different way of moving in the
world—that the world was basically okay, as long as we didn't mess with it
too much, that living in harmony with the Way was more important than
worldly striving. Lao-tzu taught accomplishing without doing, the way of
letting things take their course.

183

Sometimes I wonder if this book which insinuated itself so deeply
into the axioms of my thought was really a positive influence. How often
had I let the way of inaction be an excuse for avoidance? Maybe I should
have stayed with Camus and followed the absurd. Do we really want to rely
on knotted strings rather than writing? And how traceless should a life be?

Good walking leaves no tracks . . .

Over a thousand years after Lao-tzu, the Chan master Tung Shan
taught the "Bird Path," the trackless way. Another thousand years later one
of his descendants, the Soto master Shigetsu Ein, wrote:

In extending the hands, there is no separate road; it does not transgress the
bird's path. Traveling the bird's path by yourself, yet you extend your
hands. In the bird's path there is no separate road; knowing the hidden
roads yourself, you still don't transgress it. Dwelling in the bird's path,
you don't sprout horns on your head but always extend your hands.

Picking and choosing.
Shouting secrets.
Painting tracks on the wall.

Leaving messages.

Quotations taken from the following books:
Cleary, Thomas, and J. C. Cleary, *The Blue Cliff Record,* Shambhala, 1992.
MacHovec, Frank J., tr., *The Book of Tao,* Peter Pauper Press, 1962.
Powell, William F., *The Record of Tung-shan,* University of Hawaii, 1986.
Red Pine, tr., *Lao-Tzu's Taoteching,* Mercury House, 1996.

Poet **Dale Pendell** is the author of *Pharmako/Poeia: Plant Powers, Poisons, and Herbcraft,* and *Pharmako/Dynamis: A Guide for Adepts.* He produces "Leaf Songs, Invocations of Plant Allies," with the Oracular Madness Choir and studies Zen at the Ring of Bone Zendo in northern California.

Knowledge is structured in consciousness.

MAHARISHI MAHESH YOGI

❖

MICHAEL BARNARD

The Infinite Well

IN 1971, I HAD THE GOOD FORTUNE TO BECOME THE FILMMAKER FOR MAHARISHI Mahesh Yogi (the founder of Transcendental Meditation). I had been attending, along with two thousand others, a teacher-training course in Mallorca, Spain. This course originally had been slated to take place in Rishikesh, India, but due to the unexpectedly large number of people wanting to become teachers of Transcendental Meditation, the course organizers had scrambled to find enough inexpensive hotel rooms to house us all. Winters on Mallorca meant a lot of empty hotel rooms, so there we were, meditating twelve hours a day for three months, while our northeast-facing edge of the island took the brunt of endless Mediterranean winter storms— assaults that echoed the earlier invasions by Moors, North Africans, and assorted pirates.

The locals accepted this invasion of two thousand young people mostly from America, Germany, and England with a resigned equanimity. And why not? We were a new breed of winter tourists who never went outside and who didn't even *want* a good steak and fine wine!

Near the end of our course, each of us had a personal meeting with Maharishi in which he would ask why we wanted to be teachers. During my interview, as he looked at my résumé, he noticed that I had earned an advanced degree and that I made films. Never mind that my degree was an

MFA in painting and that my avant garde, experimental films were seen and appreciated by only rarified aesthetes. He suggested that I stay on and make films for him and start an entire film department. The pay would be room, board, and twenty-five dollars a month. And I, with my Bolex camera, my MFA, a pregnant (and unbelievably tolerant) wife, and no money in the bank, instantly agreed.

We went home seven years later. In the meantime, we followed Maharishi across Europe and North America several times, eventually building an actual film production facility in an old Borscht Belt hotel in the Catskills. During that seven years we saw the small, charmingly Indian-style informal organization grow, as Transcendental Meditation became a media-driven craze in the United States and abroad. And, in the course of all this travel and change, we began to know Maharishi and the teachings behind the simple technique known to the world as TM.

This technique of meditation is deceptively simple and is entirely based on Vedic knowledge and tradition. One of the things that attracted me to TM was that it had no particular religious affiliation and no requirement to be part of a group for the practice to be effective. Indeed, I have had little connection with the TM movement for over twenty years, yet I practice the meditation twice a day and am ever more thankful that I began this practice when I did.

Maharishi Mahesh Yogi, repeating the phrase, "Knowledge is structured in consciousness," reminded us of the essential nature of life and how our meditation practice was bringing us into harmony with that blissful natural state where pure consciousness is integrated with the relative states of existence. Ultimately, through repeated transcending during meditation, the nervous system becomes habituated to that field of pure awareness and spontaneously maintains it even during waking, dreaming, and sleeping.

"Knowledge is structured in consciousness" is an ancient Vedic formula that shows how one's state of consciousness entirely affects one's experience and thus one's knowledge. If you happen to be wearing rose-tinted glasses, the world appears rose-colored. In the same way, if your mind is clear, the world is experienced clearly. If your mind is established in pure consciousness then your experience of the world is utterly expanded and clarified. If your mind is not so clear, it is like being ill with the flu: the world is experienced in a limited, painful way. Plainly, you are not getting all of life's potential at that moment! Yet, when health returns, your experience opens up like the sun rising and your mind is clearer, happier, and more powerful. So it is when we establish our mind in pure awareness, the rest of our experience is opened up and we become spontaneously more creative.

It was exactly thirty years ago that I set out with my newly pregnant wife to TM teacher training in Mallorca. As with any life, much water has flowed under the bridge during those thirty years. There have been turbulent eddies and serene, slow-flowing episodes. My children have grown and had their own children; my wife and I have gone our amicably separate ways. And through it all I have continued my practice of meditating each day, morning and evening, rarely missing a session. Why would I do that? Is it, as some have suggested, a psychological crutch, a New Age cop-out? Or is it something more substantial?

I have been reluctant to speak publicly about my inner life. It is intensely private and lively. What I will say is that I have gained, and continue to gain, great mental clarity and inner calmness. This inner clarity and familiarity with the deeper workings of my thought process has allowed for some revelatory experiences and understandings. Many of these tend toward the area of life most commonly called "religious." There is so much confusion and misunderstanding around religion, and what constitutes religious experience at present, that a useful discussion of that subject is probably beyond the scope of this writing. Suffice it to say that my experience of the fundamentally spiritual nature of reality has only grown over the years. It doesn't much matter what these experiences are, but they are of a nature and quality that indicates most decisively the vast potential of the human race if we would access this truly astounding aspect of ourselves.

My investigation becomes subtler here, because much of what I have experienced through meditation has to do with a realm that could easily be seen as magical—the deepest area of thinking known in the Veda as *Rhitam Para Pragyah,* or, as Maharishi likes to call it: The Field of All Possibilities. This is the area where the inner and the outer are one, where thoughts first manifest out of the unbounded, undefined state of pure consciousness. It is precisely this area that becomes more and more familiar as we develop our consciousness, as we quiet the noise in our mind and begin to see what is actually there. For me, a student with much to learn, just seeing this jewel of dynamic, creative consciousness glimmering in the distance is a call to keep going, to know that more lies ahead in my own personal journey. We all get a taste of the future's possibilities from time to time. Learning to recognize and then act wisely on these snippets of inspiration is a fundamental skill all seekers must develop. I have learned that teachers come to us when we are *really* ready for them and not a moment sooner. They come in every size, shape, age, and predisposition. We only have to pay attention and gratefully accept the teachings being given to us. We only have to gracefully give back when we are able.

Most people in today's frenetic world live with an incredible amount of inner noise, their minds awash with surging, criss-crossing currents of psychic static to the point where the notion of inner silence has become an arcane, foreign concept for the general public. I, and other practitioners of meditation, can easily take for granted the experience of thoughts springing from that infinite well of inner silence in a constant recapitulation of creation, every instant of every day. It's happening all the time for everyone. We are lucky to experience this lucidly and to appreciate just how miraculous and divine existence truly is. Just for this experience, I am grateful. As with any other seeker, everything in my life is informed by this simple, basic experience.

Michael Barnard is a writer, painter, photographer, and filmmaker. He has written short stories, poetry, and feature film scripts, including *The Outermost House* and *The Transfiguration of Fast Eddie Rose.* Barnard moved to Los Angeles in 1978 and has worked on a wide variety of film and television productions.

Hello Kuan Yin, I love you.
Hello Kuan Yin, I love you.
Miao Shan, Avalokitesvara, Arya Tara
You are all to me!
Thank you for teaching me how to talk to you.
(sound the bell)
Listen, listen to the beautiful sound
It brings me back to my true home.

BARBARA J. HODGSON

BARBARA J. HODGSON

Being Truly Home

WHEN ASKED, "HOW DID YOU STEP ONTO THE BUDDHIST PATH?" MANY MEMORIES, thoughts, and ideas fly through my head. To ascertain that moment of first recognition, that first intuitive impulse that I was truly home, was a daunting exercise. I have often heard that if you are practicing Buddhism now, you have practiced it before and probably for a number of lifetimes. I have picked up the pen so many times to answer this question, to write down my thoughts, but today I have a tingling sensation that I will succeed. I am sitting on the beach in Santa Barbara, an unusually desolate beach for such a popular place. I am ready to start, my pen is poised, the yellow pad is in my lap, and I begin to write.

One by one birds appear. They finally gain my attention as twelve of them gather in front of me, forming a half circle, a curving chorus line. I begin examining them one by one, noticing their differences. Some are black, others white and gray, and others are mottled brown. I also see the difference in their shapes and sizes. Still studying them, I begin to talk to them, explaining why I'm here and what I am trying to accomplish. They are so attentive that I want to give them something back, so I begin telling them the story of Kuan Yin and the peacock.

In the beginning of time, as the story goes, Kuan Yin lived with the creatures on the earth. She taught them how to live together happily and how to show kindness to their young. But one day, she told them she would be ascending into heaven to take up her commitments there. The animals were devastated when they heard this. They begged her to stay. But Kuan Yin knew she had to leave and ascended to heaven on a cloud.

The creatures left behind were brokenhearted. Soon arguments started, then anger and jealousy broke out among them. They became ferocious and attacked one another. Weaker ones had to run or hide from the stronger ones. Kuan Yin heard the noise, and looking down, she saw the confusion. She descended to earth immediately and asked them, "Why can't you live together in peace? Each of you has your own place and role, so why are you so envious of each other? Why can't you live in equanimity? My friends, it is obvious that I cannot be with you at all times to watch over you."

Suddenly, she swept her hands across her face and then spread them over a big bird with dull brown feathers. Instantly the bird exploded in color and light so bright that the other creatures had to turn away. But when they finally looked back, they saw a bird with one hundred tail feathers and on each of the feathers was a bright clear eye looking at them. "I cannot watch over you at all times and in all places," Kuan Yin explained, "but the peacock can. Each of his eyes will watch over you and guard you so when you see the peacock's hundred eyes you will know that I care for all of you."

Still gazing at the birds, I begin to chant mantras to them: *"Om tare tuttare ture soha"* comes first, Tara's chant. I sing it over and over. Then, I sing the Avalokitesvara chant: *"Om mani peme hung."* After a while I stop chanting and begin to meditate. One by one, the birds fly off. Looking at the waves of the Pacific, stretching out on a sandy beach, feeling the grains run through my fingers and toes, I perceive the connectedness of all living things. Happy to share my space and heart with these birds, I smile and think, "Kuan Yin is very happy."

I first met Kuan Yin in San Francisco's Chinatown. Walking into the Canton Bazaar, I was in hot pursuit of a Foo dog. What color, what size, what material, I did not know, but I knew I'd find it. My partner was with me and said, "Come here, you've got to see this!" He had found a rather large Foo dog, and it had company. There was a lady seated on top of him. She was sitting very straight, with gentle yet penetrating eyes, holding a scroll in her right hand. I later learned that the name of her posture is "Royal Ease."

A sales clerk walked up, extending her hand. "Hello, I am Pita and this is Kuan Yin, the goddess of love and mercy. She is sitting on a Foo dog which is an emblem of value and energy, a complement of wisdom. She is from a temple." Pita placed her hand on the arched tail of the dog. "You can see it is carved out of a single piece of wood, and at one time it was completely painted, but now only some of the color remains, which tells you it is a very old statue." I loved it but winced at the cost. My friend pulled out a couple of large bills and said, "You have to have this treasure; here is my contribution."

Pita continued, "Princess Miao Shan, the earthly manifestation of Kuan Yin, was so kind and loving that she was given the name Maiden with the Heart of the Buddha. But Miao Shan's life was not easy, for she pursued the life of a nun instead of the life of a princess in the palace. She had to face many hardships and endure much suffering, but her acts of compassion and love prevailed in every difficult situation until . . ." Pita made a wave with her hands, "until she became a Buddha." When I heard these words I was shocked. An ordinary human being can become a Buddha? I had always thought there was only one Buddha, like there is only one God. I was speechless at the possibility that a human being could become transformed, become enlightened, and become a Buddha. Kuan Yin had done it!

"Kuan Yin has such an appeal," said Pita, "since she responds to the heartfelt needs of ordinary people. She is the friend you call upon in times of trouble, the hand that guides you. She does not reveal any new philosophy or truth, for she is truth. Nor does she lead initiates into deep mysteries of meditation; you just talk to her. Meditate in front of her, and the answers and the truth will come. Just talk to her." I thanked the saleswoman.

The transaction was complete and reality overtook the story. How do we get her home? "No problem, she can fit in the back seat of the car," Brian assured me. We went off to get the car, thoroughly amazed at what had just happened. We placed her carefully on the back seat, tightened the seat belt around her, and headed back to Los Angeles. Every now and then, I looked over my shoulder to see if she was still there. The statue seemed oddly real; I sensed a powerful presence emanating from it.

When we arrived home, it was late at night, but we quickly started rearranging the bedroom furniture until we found just the right spot for Kuan Yin. However, I was disappointed to see her on the floor. Brian is a craftsman and he quickly reassured me that he would build a proper stand for her. I was greatly relieved; I knew this would be my new altar. Over the next few weeks, I started meditating in front of her and took Pita's suggestion to "just talk to her." The time I spent was shorter than my usual meditation practice. I felt such power and energy from her and so many thoughts and pictures streamed through my head, that I was a little afraid.

One morning when I was meditating at dawn, looking at the statue's beautiful face, I suddenly remembered the fall of my senior year in high school. Dinner was over and I was ready to race out with my friends. Run-around-Sue would be there in a matter of minutes. Mom said, "Oh, no you don't. We must read from the *Upper Room* and pray first." I agreed to say the prayer, hoping to get it over with sooner. My dad, a minister, read the scripture and devotion in somber tones. Then it was my turn to say the prayer, which I wasn't used to doing, but I had to in order to take off with the gang. I started praying in a jerky, hesitant style. All of a sudden I felt an incredible sensation of love and bliss flood through my sixteen-year-old body. Words started coming out of my mouth about love and that the only important thing in this human life is compassion and mercy. My yearning voice called for people to love one another, to be kind to one another, and to resolve their differences; to replace strife, jealousy, and hatred with peace, kindness, and love. Compassion welled up in me, a kind of love I had never felt before.

When the prayer was over, the rest of my family disappeared quietly. I was sitting there in the kitchen filled with bliss, love, and joy, with no desire to run off and cruise Woodward Avenue with my friends. I remembered that incredible feeling—feeling beyond words—lasting for a very long time. As the vividness of the memory began to dim, I returned my awareness to the meditation cushion and looked up at Kuan Yin's face. Distinctly I heard her say, "That was me!"

Gratefully, I thank the lovely ladies of Chinatown for their stories of Kuan Yin and especially for my teacher and friend Dagmola (Sakya Dagmo Kusho), who is the emanation of Kuan Yin Arya Tara.

Barbara J. Hodgson, a communications consultant based in Los Angeles, develops and implements public relations and creative marketing campaigns for clients focusing on life-enhancing issues: health, the environment, human rights, and other cause-related efforts. Her two daughters, Vanessa and Nicole, live in San Francisco. Hodgson is a Tibetan Buddhist practitioner and is the director of the Mother Tara Sakya Center, Tara-Ling, founded in Los Angeles by her teacher Sakya Dagmo Kusho. The Center's Web page is www.TaraLing.com.

The milk of grace overflows in torrents to the loving heart,
to the thirsty and yearning soul.
Childlike innocence, pure and sincere love
attract the milk of grace.

BABA NARD SINGH JI MAHARAJ

SURINDER MANN

The Front Room

I WONDER IF IT IS THE SAME FOR ALL FAMILIES?

I wonder whether everyone's parents get so tired of all their favorite possessions getting scratched, torn, or broken that they decide to make their own demilitarized zone—a special room for their special material things. My dad kept the front room of our home in London off limits to all his six kids. There he kept the nice sofa, the color TV, and the hi-fi. There the walls had pictures in frames, not just calendars that came with pictures on the top half of the fold.

Sometimes my father would let us in the room, especially if there were guests present, as it was for them that the room was really intended. In we would come: my twin sister, my younger brother, and me. The other three kids were either too young to appreciate the treat or not yet born. There we would watch TV, seeing the colors change in *The Wizard of Oz,* and there we would see cartoons as they were meant to be seen. The TV screen even had a kind of magnifying glass in front of it to make the image larger, only you had to watch the screen head on; from the side the picture looked like gasoline on a puddle, all the colors swirling. I remember the day the door-to-door salesman came and my dad bought it.

There was something else about the room, though, that had us puzzled. There were pictures in the white band above the wallpaper that separated the ceiling from the walls, and the pictures were all of quite bloody scenes

201

that involved Sikhs[1] dead or dying. One picture had a Sikh being boiled alive. The three of us studied it and eventually asked our father to explain why such violent pictures were on the front-room wall.

Our father described how four hundred years ago the Muslim rulers of Kashmir had conducted a campaign to force all Hindus to convert to Islam. The Hindu leaders turned to the Sikh Guru for help. The Guru, after listening to their stories, declared that if he could be converted, then all would be converted. He journeyed to Dehli to meet the emperor but was immediately arrested. First the emperor ordered him placed on a hot iron plate and burning sand poured over him. Then he was boiled in water, after which he was finally drowned. Not once through this ordeal did he renounce his faith.

Hearing this, the three of us were quiet, quieter than young children normally are. It was our first knowledge that cruelty existed beyond our own small concerns. Suddenly we were transported out of the front room and into violent and bloody times. We could imagine water so hot that it burned and the pain of it, but we could not imagine a will so strong that it defied it. So we quickly moved on to our next game.

Our father had sat on the edge of a sofa and quietly told us of the faith of his fathers. We were now small children framed by a much larger story, one that was burned into my memory. Years later I would ask myself how anyone could be so cruel; how could anyone watch someone be tortured so and not end it with compassion? Where did such disregard and lack of empathy come from? Sadly, years have only brought more horrors that have been committed in our own times. The antidote, though, has always been the picture of a man being tortured to death but showing no fear and no pain because he knew his example would prevail.

The picture is still there, only now next to it hangs one of my father. And now the story is mine to tell.

---

[1] Sikhism is a more recent faith that grew out of a rethinking of the relationship between peoples as defined by Hinduism and Islam. It sought to address the inequality that the caste system had produced while allowing for freedom of beliefs. Sikhs are predominantly found in the north of India but have settled throughout the world.

Surinder Mann's father and mother migrated from the Punjab in India to England in the 1960s. His family has never returned to India. He is one of six children. For the past six years he has been working as a structural engineer in Los Angeles and Milwaukee.

When the door is shut, what builds is heat and pressure.
And heat and pressure are the soil of growth.
In that heat, the flower of freedom blooms.

JOKO BECK

◈

JOKO BECK

The Key

AN INTERESTING DEFINITION OF FREEDOM IS: "FREEDOM IS WHEN THERE AIN'T nothing to lose." Naturally, we all wish to be free. To be free is to realize what wisdom and compassion are. This freedom is the jewel of our practice—it is what we are seeking, here, there, everywhere; and what we often fail to see is that our life, just as it is, is the jewel. Whenever I say this, someone invariably will say, "She must be kidding!" But the Four Noble Truths tell us that life is suffering, there is a cause to suffering, and there is a way out of suffering, to freedom. We forget these truths and where they point.

Let's look for a moment at our usual way of viewing freedom: freedom is being able to do what I want, what I like; to be able to go where I wish, to be where I want to be; to live life as I choose to live it. And if something interferes with my wishes, I say: "My freedom is threatened." We usually view freedom in this way.

To keep our "freedom," we are anxious to leave a little loophole in any involvement. We sense our uneasiness if our escape route is blocked. The fact is that to preserve our so-called freedom, we always try to leave a door open so we can escape.

Closely connected with understanding freedom is another word, one that is even stickier for most of us. It is *commitment*. As we practice, as we do *zazen,* what we discover is a subtle lack of commitment to anything or anyone; as we sit, we encounter our schemes, our fancies, our manipulative tricks. And practice is the process of wearing out (by seeing, by making conscious) the hundreds of ways we have of leaving that door open, of staying uncommitted to anything—our practice, another person, our work—because it's true, isn't it, that "nothing should threaten my freedom; and if it does, I'll be on my way, thank you, out the door!"

Freedom is also closely connected with two words we have often talked about, *pain* and *suffering.* The dictionary may say that pain and suffering are the same. But in the way we are using them, suffering is the running out the door, the escaping; pain, which is the other side of joy, is to stay and commit to being in the experience of life as it is. Pain/joy: interchangeable. So how can we turn suffering into joy?

We turn it by understanding commitment. When we commit ourselves, we give totally and hold nothing back. Nothing. No door is left open out of which to escape. Now I don't want to be misunderstood—not all relationships have reached a stage where they should be committed. Commitment is, of course, frightening because of our fears of being hurt; fear exists in each one of us. But *until* we shut the door—which is our desire to escape—only then can we sense *who* is running; *who* is suffering; *who* feels caught—*who we are.*

The last thing that appeals to us is to shut the door. So how can we do it? How do we commit ourselves? We just sit. Motionless and silent, we face up to what our life is: pain is okay, weariness is okay, confusion is okay. We shut the door to our wish to escape from all that. And what is the difference between most relationships and marriage (even though not all marriages are committed)? Nearly always in relationships we leave the door open a crack; in a true marriage, we shut the door. We give up our ideas about freedom.

When the door is shut, what builds is heat and pressure. And heat and pressure are the soil of growth. In that heat, the flower of freedom blooms. We could say that in our practice what we must do is marry ourselves. This "I," who wants to be separate from everything else, has to meet the "I" who is everything. When we sit in *zazen* with no doors open, little by little without anyone telling us, we know that all externals are nothing but "I." And then from whom would we run?

We begin to realize that most of us are not concerned with real freedom; we are interested in escape. "Yes, I'll sit every day; well, maybe." Or "I'll stay with this person—at least until I see if I'm pleased. And even if I stay, I'll peek out of the door now and then just to be sure I'm not missing something." "I'm committed to my parents or my children or my friends—but I have to be a little careful. I don't want my freedom interfered with." Are we committed?

Even more serious is that we don't commit ourselves to ourselves. We *always* leave a door open. "I'll sit tomorrow. I'll do *sesshin* some other time." There are multiple, continuous ways in which we escape from our lives; we even dream of enlightenment. But there is no dream in enlightenment, only what is, and our commitment to it. From what would we escape if all eyes are this eye? What to escape from?

Many people feel that they are going through difficult times. But in a sense, times are only difficult because we think they should be otherwise. We haven't shut the door. We don't see that true freedom is to commit ourself to the pain and pressure of our life—just to experience what is—and "cook." What do we get when we cook? Can you answer?

Charlotte Joko Beck is a Zen teacher and the head of the San Diego Zen Center. In the 1960s she trained under Hakuun Yasutani Roshi and Soen Nakagawa Roshi. In 1983 she became the Third Dharma heir of Hakuyu Maezumi Roshi of the Zen Center of Los Angeles. She is the author of two books, *Everyday Zen: Love and Work* and *Nothing Special: Living Zen.*

May I accomplish the profound path of transference into the pure land.
May I gain the rainbow body through Buddha's blessings.
May I become inseparable from the heart-mind of Kyanrazig.

FROM THE *P'HOWA* PRAYER

CYNTHIA LESTER

Death, Not Death

IN MY YOUNG ADULTHOOD I BECAME A SPIRITUAL COUNSELOR. BECAUSE OF MY clairvoyant abilities, which I was working to refine, it was not uncommon for me to see people's souls in various states of transition. I later became a Tibetan Buddhist and received the teaching of *P'howa,* the transference of consciousness at the time of death. The teaching is given to a practitioner by a high lama, known as a Tulku, in the form of an empowerment. The teaching describes in detail the signs of approaching death and gives instructions for what to do at the moment of passing. The prayer, which is many pages long, is meant to help the dying person leave the body.

Whenever I am feeling overcome by grief or anger at the seeming unfairness of death, there are three lines I repeat to myself: "May I accomplish the profound path of transference into the pure land. May I gain the rainbow body through Buddha's blessings. May I become inseparable from the heart-mind of Kyanrazig." Before I received the *P'howa* teaching, I attempted in my own way to connect passing souls with some kind of image or vision that would help them move away from their physical bodies. With *P'howa* I had specific instructions directly from the teachings of the Buddha.

One of my dear friends was killed in a car crash many years ago. On the evening following her death, I felt her confusion and sorrow at being separated from her body and her husband. I could hear her crying out to her husband, "Mickey, Mickey, what happened?" Since I knew she was a woman of strong spiritual faith, I prayed the *P'howa* to her: "May I accomplish the profound path of transference into the pure land. May I gain the rainbow body through Buddha's blessings. May I become inseparable from the heart-mind of Kyanrazig." What a great comfort to offer the concept of pure lands, a light body, and Kyanrazig—the Tibetan Buddha of compassion. In sudden deaths, both the departing soul and family and friends may experience much confusion about what has happened and what to do. It is an honor for me to be able to assist them by sharing this ancient technique.

In our current era of AIDS and cancer, victims of these diseases and their families often experience the gradual unfolding of death. Watching the body slowly deteriorate and lose its life force helps us to accept the soul's departure. *P'howa* assures people of the continuity of all souls, as well as the soul's ability to consciously leave the body while it stays focused on choosing the next step of infinite existence.

When my dear friend of many years was struggling to keep her tiny, cancer-ravaged body alive, I shared the *P'howa* prayer with her. I hoped it would ease her pain and give her a new vision and healing while reminding her that death is a transference, not an end. Sharing the ritual of *P'howa* with grieving family members also lets them participate in the transition and gain a deeper understanding of the great illusion of death. *P'howa* reminds us that dying consciously is actually something we practice all our lives. Every step involves birth, life, death, and rebirth to a new experience.

I have followed many beloved friends and clients through the soul's transition. Death always comes as a surprise even when we know it is coming. The *P'howa* teachings help me set aside my grief, as well as the grief of the others left behind, so that I can help the transitioning soul leave us freely, with our blessings. We thus help one another to become more conscious of our physical state and to fly free of the body vessel when its journey is done. The soul's journey never ends.

Cynthia Lester has been an intuitive counselor and teacher for twenty-five years as well as a Buddhist. She lives in Tucson, Arizona. Her Web site is www.cynthialester.com.

Gate gate paragate, parasamgate bodhi svaha.

FROM THE *HEART SUTRA*

✦

Every little thing's gonna be all right.

BOB MARLEY

✦

GRACE BRUMETT

Gone Beyond: A Question of Letting Go

WHY DOESN'T HE JUST DIE! WHY CAN'T IT ALL BE OVER? IT IS HARD TO EXPLAIN now how I could utter such desperate thoughts even as my heart was breaking. The man I loved lay before me, his body ravished by cancer but his piercing blue eyes steady and true as ever. Death had not yet arrived, even after five arduous years on the battlefront, in and out of every conceivable treatment and hospital ward.

My little family felt as though it was bound together on a raft, that was barreling down a fierce and wild canyon river. The rapids tossed and tore at us. We received small respite in the infrequent eddies called "remission," yet we all knew the giant falls were ahead, and one of us would not come out alive. We didn't know when, but we knew without doubt this time would arrive. There was nothing we could do but hang on.

My practice became that of patient acceptance and blind faith. The words of Bob Marley—"Every little thing's gonna be all right"—became my mantra. It's easy to confuse faith and trust with passivity, but they are not the same. Sometimes things occur in life which we simply cannot change. We can only choose how we want to go through them.

Why *couldn't* he just die? Was our great love for him holding him back rather than releasing him? I'd had plenty of practice with letting go along the way, knowing from my long years of Buddhist practice that all things

change, and there is nothing to which one can truly cling. I had watched
while we lost our business, our good credit, and even our home. Many times
I had chanted from the Heart Sutra, "*Gate gate paragate, parasamgate bodhi
svaha.*" (Gone, gone, gone beyond. Gone completely beyond. Form is no
other than emptiness. Emptiness is no other than form.) I thought I understood what that meant. I had watched Michael lose his sense of who he
was—or was not. One by one they slipped away: his health—he is not that;
his good looks—he is not that; his role as provider, as lover—not that. Until
we knew that he was none of these. None of them mattered. Stripped of
these roles and identifications, he became more and more who he truly
was—his essential self. Yet, now we both had to face this biggest and most
real of losses. He was about to leave his body. How do I let go of this man
I have loved for twenty-five years who fathered my three children?

In his last week Michael had stopped eating and the pain was growing
worse. The tumor at the top of his spine threatened to paralyze him.
Michael would look at me in stark terror. "This cannot go on. It must end."
He needed release from his incredibly strong body. But how? I called my
friend Tisha, a Buddhist and healer.

"Get him to a lama."

She knew of one in Corralitos. I called.

"I must see a lama. I must see Lama Tarchang immediately."

"I'm sorry. It's impossible. There is a lama retreat now. They cannot be
interrupted or reached for the entire month."

"That will be too late. This is urgently important. My husband is
dying, and he *must* see a lama before it's too late."

"I'll call you back."

She did. "Okay, Lama Tarchang says he will see you. Can you be here
at noon?"

"Yes."

I called a close friend. "Will you come along to help? What should
I take?"

We bought a small bottle of the very best whiskey and a traditional
white silk blessing scarf. I picked some flowers from my garden, and we
were off.

Michael was very frail and easy to lift into the wheelchair; this giant of a man who had once swung chain saws over his back so easily and run up and down steep mountainsides all day. We drove off to the lama, not knowing what to expect but intuitively sensing that he held a key. It was such a lovely summer day, fragrant and heady and alive. Michael was animated. With his morphine patch in place, straw hat on his bony, gray chemo head, he talked nonstop as we slowly went the back route past houses he had proudly built. The road began to twist and climb through redwoods and over noisy little creeks. And then we were there.

The woman at the office was impersonal and businesslike. In her role as protector of the center she was ready to shoo us away.

"We're here to see Lama Tarchang."

"I'm sorry. He is in retreat."

"I know. But he said he would see us. My husband, Michael Brumett, is outside."

"Oh, yes." She seemed to recognize the name, or at least the urgency in my voice.

"Wait there across the meadow by that building."

I wheeled Michael over like a mother hen, triumphant and determined. The sun was warm. Michael had the whiskey and blessing scarf. We sat in the delicious sunshine redolent with butterflies and buzzing bees. And then a small man in a maroon robe with his long hair tied in a knot on top of his head and a wide grin on his face suddenly came around the corner. Casual and unpretentious, he sat down knee to knee with Michael.

"Hello, Michael."

"I like your hair," Michael replied, equally unpretentious and honest, meaning no disrespect.

Lama Tarchang laughed and showed him how the knot of hair was wound so carefully.

Michael gave him the gifts.

"Well, Michael . . ."

Without hesitation, Michael looked directly at him.

"I'm ready to go."

"Ah, well, no big deal."

And then he began to describe it, what it would be, how it would be. Exactly. Beautifully.

"Nothing wrong you can do . . . just release surrounded by peace and love . . . you are Buddha . . . go into the clear sky . . . all love . . . to heaven, nirvana. It is called many things. . . . I am so happy I can meet you in this form. Things don't just happen by chance. . . . I will pray for you for forty-nine days. . . ." He touched Michael gently on the forehead and told him he loved him.

"I don't want my family to worry about me."

Lama Tarchang turned to me with a few instructions. And like a schoolgirl I took note of all the details. I wanted it right. We were coming very near, and there would be no more dress rehearsals.

Holding my hand, with quiet gentle words he told me, "This transition is perfectly natural and normal. In a hundred years all life here will be gone. Be calm. Send only love and peace to him to help. As he goes, touch only the top of his head."

And then Michael asked a final question. "I want to be clear when I go. I have this morphine patch. I don't want to be drugged." He was a student, too.

The lama laughed. "Instant out of body, instant clear. There is nothing to fear. It is perfectly safe."

I'm sure he was right. I trust these lamas know about that part. Michael knows now, now that it is all over. What *I* know is that we went home from there and Michael held our hands—he and I and our three children—in a last circle, not letting go. Then he climbed the stairs all by himself, hoisting his body up with his arms, as his leg was broken—stubborn man that he always was.

Two days later I looked directly, deeply into those eyes and kept my promise. "It's okay to go. I am fine. The children are fine. We can do this together. My love is with you always forever." We breathed together one last breath, and off he went, just like that. He grew bigger and bigger. He filled the room and beyond. Finally free. No big deal. And yet the biggest deal of all.

218

Six months after he died, I held his ashes before tossing them into the sea, and I pondered once again, *"Gate gate paragate parasamgate bodhi svaha."* (Form is no other than emptiness, emptiness is no other than form.) If this is not you—and it definitely is not—then who are you? What and where is the essence of *you* that transcends this ash matter, this crushed bone? The consciousness that moved this matter, the life and the awareness really 219 didn't die. It simply went beyond form. With nowhere to go, it is just as present as ever. I can feel it.

Now, with so much letting go done, I simply cannot use the word *loss* to adequately describe what happened. Nothing is really ever lost when you let it go. My love remains the same, and Michael's love didn't go away either. It's just different. And every little thing is truly all right.

Grace Brumett was a student of Robert Aitken Roshi and a member of Ring of Bone Zendo for several years. During that time she was the private literary secretary for Gary Snyder. Brumett spent fifteen years as a teacher. She is a published writer and currently works as a freelance editor. She lives on a wooden sailboat in Mexico.

Even Bhagavan, the supreme Lord,
during those autumn nights,
having gazed upon
blooming jasmine flowers,
turned his mind
toward love's delights,
fully taking refuge in
Yogamaya's magic powers.

BHAGAVATA PURANA

GRAHAM M. SCHWEIG

Beauty Captures Devotee and Divinity

SEVERAL YEARS AGO, WHEN WRITING MY DOCTORAL DISSERTATION. I FOUND myself transported by the exquisite passages of Sanskrit poetic verse found in one of the most revered sacred texts in all India, the *Bhagavata Purana*. The comeliness of the verse was striking. Within this sacred text, embedded in sounds, rhythms, and meanings of words, were glimpses of the divine beauty of God's world.

In India, the vision of God is hardly that of Ezekiel's biblical revelation of a divine throne with daunting power and overwhelming might from which a blinding light emanates, rendering it virtually inaccessible. Rather, the supreme Lord, Krishna, whose flute music entrances all beings, is described as having the beautiful, bluish figure of a young boy. He is a playful cowherd who delights in roaming the paradisal countryside of his divine abode called Vraja.

Indeed, the beauty of Krishna's captivating world expressed in these verses enticed me to translate Sanskrit poetry into English. On one hand, these attractive verses enhanced my dissertation; on the other, they would sometimes distract me from it. I translated these delightfully distracting verses, which conveyed to me something of the loveliness of God's surroundings and intimate play with his dearest friends and family, from various parts of the *Bhagavata*'s famous tenth book.

Thus, a gentle breeze
from the clear waters of autumn
carries sweet scents of lotus flowers.
Entering that pleasing scene
with cows and cowherd friends,
Acyuta [Krishna, "the infallible one"] appears.

Among groves of flowering trees
swarming with maddened bees,
and lakes, rivers and hills
resounding with flocks of birds,
Madhupati [Krishna] enters with Balarama
and the cowherd boys.

BHAGAVATA PURANA 10.21.1–2

These are the two opening verses of the chapter known as the *Venu Gita*, the "Song of the Flute." It is characteristic for the author of this text to describe the natural imagery and sounds of this perfect world in poetically rich language, as an introduction to the divine Krishna who plays his flute, enlivened by the sublime setting. The performance is stunning, and all who hear it feel their hearts melting:

While tending his cows
he began to sound his flute.
Gazing upon Krishna,
whose beauty and personality
is a festival for all women,
and hearing enchanting music
emanating from his flute,
the hearts of celestial goddesses
moving in air ships
are shaken by passion.
They become bewildered

as their belts loosen
and flowers fall from their hair.

Then cows drink the nectar
of the song of the flute
flowing from Krishna's mouth
into vessels of their up-raised ears.
Calves stand still, indeed,
their mouths filled with milk
flowing from their mothers' nipples.
Watching with tearful eyes,
they embrace Govinda [Krishna]
within their hearts.

O mother, these birds in the forest
are very likely great sages
who have seen Krishna,
whose melodious flute song
has elevated them all.
Rising to branches of trees
with beautiful foliage,
these birds listen
with closed eyes
while all other voices vanish.

When rivers hear the music of Mukunda [Krishna]
their flowing currents are broken
and their waters begin to swirl
because of intense feelings for him.
The two feet of Murari [Krishna],
becoming stationary
while embraced by armlike waves,
are seized while offerings
of lotus flowers are made.

BHAGAVATA PURANA 10.21.12–15

Indeed, so enchanting a place is this heavenly Vraja that God is utterly moved toward love. I find no better expression of this than in the very first verse of the famous Rasalila ("Dance of Divine Love") within the *Bhagavata Purana*:

226

Even Bhagavan, the supreme Lord,
during those autumn nights,
having gazed upon
blooming jasmine flowers,
turned his mind
toward love's delights,
fully taking refuge in
Yogamaya's magic powers.

BHAGAVATA PURANA 10.29.1

The unparalleled beauty of the Vraja scenery builds in the next verse, inspiring the divine soloist to create sweet music on his flute and alluring young milk maidens who run off to accompany him:

Seeing lotus flowers bloom
and the perfect circle of the moon,
whose light is like the face of the goddess Rama
reddish like fresh kumkuma,
then seeing the forest colored
by the moon's gentle rays,
he began to make sweet music
entrancing young maidens with beautiful eyes.

Upon hearing such sweet music
increasing their love,
the young women of Vraja
whose minds were captured by Krishna,
unaware of one another,

went off to the place
where their beloved was waiting,
with their earrings swinging wildly.

BHAGAVATA PURANA 10.29.3–4

The message, embodied in exquisite Sanskrit verse, is clear. The divine   *227*
realm is filled with paradisal beauty stimulating loving passion for God
and his devotees. Thus, God himself is capable of becoming captivated by
such natural opulence and sublime scenery. This God of India is a deity of
intimacy who entrances souls by an unsurpassed ambiance and intoxicat-
ing music, creating a heaven of the heart—a truly unique contribution of a
divine aesthetic to theologies the world over.

When I was struggling to write my doctoral dissertation, the natural
beauty of these verses lifted my spirit into a realm I had never before experienced. To this day, I remember how I was transported, completely drawn
from this world by the wonder portrayed through the Rasalila's sacred
poetry, a veritable threshold to the spiritual world. The very first verse of
the passage especially captured my heart and mind, particularly the
thought that even God, the embodiment and source of all beauty, is carried
away by the splendor of his own surroundings.

Graham M. Schweig received his doctorate in comparative religion from Harvard University and is presently
Assistant Professor of Philosophy and Religious Studies at Christopher Newport University, on the Virginia
peninsula. Although Western born, he has been a practitioner of various forms of meditational and devotional yoga under the guidance of traditional teachers. Schweig has published and continues to write on
devotional yoga for scholarly anthologies and journals, encyclopedias, and academic presses.

As a bee seeks nectar from all kinds of flowers
seek teachings everywhere.
Like a deer that finds a quiet place to graze
seek seclusion to digest all that you have gathered.
Like a mad one beyond all limits
go where you please and live like a lion
completely free of all fear.

DZOGCHEN TANTRA

KEVIN KREIGER

Into the Deep

AFTER LONG ENCOURAGEMENT FROM TWO CLOSE FRIENDS, ONE OF WHOM happened to be a yoga teacher, for the first time I enrolled in some beginning yoga classes. Shortly thereafter, I threw myself into the deep end by going on a four-day yoga retreat. Talk about being in over my head! There were thirty-five yogis and yoginis, and everyone but three of us was fairly advanced. I had never even heard of, much less practiced, the vast majority of what we did that weekend. I was pushed to my limits as I had rarely been in my life.

During the second day, it happened. We were deep in yet another new pose for me, "the pigeon," and holding. My hips were screaming at being twisted in a way they'd never been before. I was struggling not to clench up and straining even more not to roll out of the position and mercifully let myself rest. Fear of staying in the posture burned through me. Fear of dropping out of it burned just as hot.

I was a novice and everyone knew it. I had every justification in the world to throw in the towel on this one. But I hadn't yet managed to embody the notion I kept hearing in class from Shiva, my teacher: Yoga is all about being wherever you are. I was there to push myself, and I was going to push! The other two beginners had long since given up on the posture. But I was going to prove to them all that I could go the distance. More than that, I was going to prove it to myself.

As I fought to contain the shakes that threatened to overcome me, Shiva's voice suddenly slipped through the haze of pain. By the time I really began to hear what she was reading, she came to the last three lines:

> *Like a mad one beyond all limits*
> *go where you please and live like a lion*
> *completely free of all fear.*

Something sparked in me. It was not a cinematic burst of determination to hold the pose, but a moment of inner quiet in which those final words kept resonating: "live like a lion, completely free of all fear." The moment seemed to dilate. I was suddenly aware of myself struggling like a fish on a hook of my own making. I was at once afraid to succeed and afraid not to succeed; afraid to admit that I was not yet expert at this new undertaking and desperately afraid of not being good enough. My ego's self-protective mechanisms were all tangled up in my head.

Perhaps more than anything else, I was very, very far from being present. My thoughts were running wild, contriving all kinds of scenarios to avoid being in the moment and facing the possibility that I was truly out of my depth, to avoid experiencing that feeling in all its fullness. I was busy trying to survive, caught in old stories of failure and pain, and projecting onto a future fantasy self who would be blissfully proficient in all the areas I was lacking. I was nowhere near the here and now.

When Shiva's voice came to me, it brought me back to the present. Reconnected to that specific moment, I felt a pulse of pure embodiment; in hindsight I will say that this was the purest yogic moment I have ever known. The need to cling to my fears vanished, and I relaxed into now. And just as I took a deep breath and knew it was time to relinquish the posture, Shiva let us out.

It is hard to explain that moment: a rush of emotion, tears in my eyes, a feeling that went far beyond the mere satisfaction of having survived the posture. I had broken through something essential, and although it would take a long time to fully process the experience, I knew that it had irrevocably changed me. The quote from the *Dzogchen,* and the context in which I encountered it, changed my life. It has become a mantra I repeat as I go through my day. When I feel fear rising, I take a deep breath and remember.

Kevin Kreiger is a screenwriter and playwright, with master's degrees in playwriting from University of California, San Diego and Shakespeare from Oxford University. He serves as a Chinese herbalist with the Tea Garden Herbal Emporium, where he is Director of the Tea Garden Institute, the Emporium's educational wing. Over the past sixteen years he has taught in numerous venues, ranging from University of California, San Diego to the Université de Bourgogne in France.

Mother of the Universe
I have no desire to exercise power.
I would not even care to be an emperor.
Sweet Mother, please grant me
Two simple meals each day,
And wealth enough to thatch the palm roof
Of my clean earthen house
Where I offer dreaming and waking
As red flowers at your feet.

RAMPRASAD

❖

ANDREW HARVEY

Honor the Sacred Feminine

IN ITS DEEPEST ESSENCE, THE DIRECT PATH IS THE PATH OF THE SACRED FEMININE because it honors at every moment the sacredness of nature, of the creation of the body, and of life itself. For the person on the Direct Path, life and universe itself are the Mother, constantly striving in both radiant and severe ways to help the human seeker to birth himself or herself into the dimension of fearless divine love and service.

On my journey into the Motherhood of God, I constantly study and meditate on texts from the *Tao Te Ching,* and the eighteenth-century Indian mother-poet Ramprasad.

The following text is taken from the twenty-eighth section of the great masterpiece of Taoism, the *Tao Te Ching.* No other mystical tradition has celebrated the humbling, nourishing, unifying powers of the sacred feminine so clearly:

> *Know the male, keep the female;*
> *Be humble toward the world.*
> *Be humble toward the world*
> *And eternal power never leaves,*
> *Returning again to innocence.*
> *Knowing the white, keep the black;*
> *Be an exemplar for the world.*

Be an exemplar for the world
And eternal power never goes awry
Returning again to infinity.
Knowing the glorious, keep the ignominious:
Be open to the world.
Be open to the world
And eternal power suffices
Returning again to simplicity.

Every line of this sublime text radiates the authentic wisdom of the Divine Feminine and helps us to live the life that can truly embody its eternal power. Lao-tzu—the author of the *Tao Te Ching*—begins this section of his masterpiece by giving us the key to the truly unified life of what I call the Direct Path:

"Know the male, keep the female."

He is telling us, "Know all the powers, forces, and passions of the male aspects of the psyche, but *keep* the female; adhere to the feminine, to sensitivity, respect, receptivity, and gentleness in all circumstances as far as possible, for the female is the course of life." Knowing the male, then, we must *keep* the female and put its powers into unforced practice if we are to be aligned with the Tao—the Mother—and always be in a position to receive the guidance and natural strength of the "root of heaven and earth."

The clue to this, as the text goes on to tell us, is in the constant unforced practice of humility. To honor the Mother always is to be always humble like Her, always serving others like Her, always considering, like Her, the holiness of others' needs and truths. Such humility exacts the highest selflessness and the cultivation of an empty "receptivity" at the core of the personality. "Be humble toward the world," Lao-tzu tells us and "eternal *power* never leaves, returning again to innocence." Humility, contrary to patriarchal designations of it as a sign of weakness, is in fact the highest imaginable sign of strength, of a realistic strength rooted in the real conditions of the body, time, and death.

Lao-tzu also tells us, it is essential to become "an exemplar for the world"—someone who is a living sign of the peace, passion, creativity, and humility of the Mother. He then goes on to reveal to us the great secret; that if such a life of service is undertaken, "eternal power never goes awry, returning again to infinity." If you have the courage to refuse the subtle temptations of transcendence, of using your mystical initiation as a way of separating yourself from the illusion of the world and enter into service as an "exemplar to the world," as a champion of love and all its powers in the real world, then you, too, will be fed directly by the healing and nourishing powers of the Mother. A life which seems initially to be *more* exhausting than the purely contemplative one will in fact turn out to be infinitely charged, infinitely nourished by the infinity of the Mother's own powers. Loving all beings with the Mother's love and putting that love into direct action and service allows anyone who does it also to drink directly from the breasts of the Mother's boundless love-energy; "an exemplar to the world" shares in the cosmic life and love energy of the Mother herself.

The key to keeping *always* nourished directly by the Mother's own infinite love-energy is, as Lao-tzu goes on to point out, "Know the glorious, keep the ignominious." If we can know the glorious—know the great visionary ecstasies of transcendence, of timeless and spaceless Divine identity—but not become obsessed with them and keep constantly the ignominious—a direct, humble, and humbling radical involvement with life in all of its holy particulars—then we will be open to the world.

Being open to the world means being open to the constant needs of others, to the pain of all beings, to the duties of championing truth, love, and justice in a crazy world. Being open to the world also means being open to the constant instruction that arrives to us from the Source through life itself. If we keep open, supple, flexible, constantly and tenderly receptive in this way, then "eternal power suffices, returning again to simplicity." We will always be filled and graced with the eternal power we need and will always be growing more and more simple with the simplicity of the Mother's own sacred passion and holiness; the eternal power we are given will suffice and will itself keep returning to that simplicity which endlessly refuels and reenergizes it.

For me, the marvelous spiritual instruction of Lao-tzu is continued and dramatized in the following mystical love song to the Mother by Ramprasad, a Hindu mystic from Bengal of the eighteenth century. No other poem I know evokes the power of the Mother on the Direct Path to transform the ordinary into the blissful, the imminent into the revelatory, and so make of the whole of life a constant dance of subtle miracle:

> *Mother of the Universe*
> *I have no desire to exercise power.*
> *I would not even care to be an emperor.*
> *Sweet Mother, please grant me*
> *Two simple meals each day,*
> *And wealth enough to thatch the palm roof*
> *Of my clean earthen house*
> *Where I offer dreaming and waking*
> *As red flowers at your feet.*
> *My green village dwelling is the abode*
> *Of your golden radiance, O Goddess.*
> *What need have I for more elaborate construction?*
> *If you surround me with the complex architecture*
> *Of stature and possession,*
> *I will refuse to call you "Mother" ever again.*
>
> *O Kali, give me just enough to serve lovingly*
> *Whatever guests may visit me.*
> *Plain metal plates and cups will do.*
> *Daily existence in the heart of my extended family*
> *Is the worship beyond worship*
> *That perceives Mother reality*
> *As every being, every situation, every breath.*
> *I will never leave this natural way of life*
> *To become a stern ascetic*

Or a teacher honored by the world.
There is only one longing this poet's soul
Declares over and over;
"Mother! Mother! Mother!
May every moment of my existence
Merge completely with your essence."

What Ramprasad is revealing to us is that an authentic life in the Mother is one of humbly incandescent simplicity, in which all the actions of all forms of awareness—both dreaming and waking—are offered as "red flowers at your feet." The real lover doesn't need any form of religious, social, or political power; nor does he or she have any need for the glamour of fame or the dominance of wealth. "Two simple meals each day" and "wealth enough to thatch the palm roof / Of my clean earthen house" are enough, and when accepted gratefully, become the normal field of a constant stream of adoration and recognition of the Mother; Ramprasad's "green village dwelling" reveals itself as the "abode of your golden radiance, O Goddess." Ordinary life, in other words—getting up, working, eating, making love, sleeping—all become conspicuously sacred experiences of the presence and grace of the Divine Mother, consciously holy ways of being with Her and thanking and celebrating and adoring Her. The whole of life becomes the consciously loved dance of Her "golden radiance."

To honor the Mother always, Ramprasad reminds us, we must keep as strongly as possible to simplicity, constantly paring down our lives to their simplest essentials. The "complex architecture of stature and possession" can all too easily blind us to Her holy presence in the smallest of everyday rituals and gestures and so blind us tragically to the sacred glory of our lives in her. Keeping simple is keeping close to the Ultimately Simple One, the Mother of all beings who has given us in life itself, when lived for and in Her, the ultimate sacred ecstasy, the Feast of Feasts.

Through honoring the Mother, the person on the Direct Path will be fed with Her eternal power, constantly refired by Her simplicity, and awakened into Her passionate love for all beings that honors every living thing.

He or she will become in and under the Mother a revolutionary of love, working at every level and in every arena of society to preserve the planet. Perhaps the deepest meaning of the Direct Path is that it is a training ground for revolutionaries of love—for beings who become empowered by the Mother's grace and passion to act in the real with her efficiency, precision, and all-transforming intensity.

Mystic and author **Andrew Harvey** was born in India and educated at Oxford. Disillusioned with academic life, he began a lifelong spiritual journey, which has shown him the importance of a direct path to God. His latest book is *The Direct Path*.

We've given up making a living.
It's all this crazy love poetry now.
It's everywhere—our eyes, our feelings,
our words—all consumed with it.

JALALUDDIN RUMI

✺

MICHAEL ATTIE

Memoirs of a Lingerie Monk

HINDUS TYPICALLY DIVIDE LIFE INTO THREE STAGES: YOUTH, HOUSEHOLDER, AND finally on retirement from a full life, spiritual seeker. In the enthusiasm of this last half-century's discovery of Eastern mysticism and meditation, my generation often reversed this progression.

This was certainly true in my case. In my twenties, I lived the life of a wandering pilgrim, staying at various monasteries and ashrams in India, Japan, and the United States. In my thirties I retired from monkhood to the "back to the land" lifestyle. I settled on a few acres in the California Sierras, built a house, and grew my own vegetables, while working at teaching and various odd jobs. At age forty, my life took another turn. My father, who was getting on in years, offered me his business, Playmates of Hollywood. If it was anything else I might have demurred, but I couldn't quite resist the prospect of owning "the world's largest lingerie store." I boarded up the cabin, headed down to L.A., and threw myself into a busy life.

At this point, I called on a Sufi sheik. I asked him, "What does it mean? Why am I going into business?" Reshad looked deep into my eyes and poured more than words into my heart: "You are going into business to give love to your customers. You may think that money and merchandise are changing hands, but that is not the important exchange. When someone leaves your store, they must feel absolutely content, like they have had a wonderful meal at the house of a most gracious host, as if they had been served hors d'oeuvres, wines, entrees, aperitifs, and desserts. They should leave feeling that every possible consideration had been made to leave nothing unsatisfied."

Then I went to my old Zen teacher, Sasaki Roshi, and asked him the same question. I got the same sort of answer: "The store is your temple. It is the center of the universe. When you know this and love being there, the customer will also love being there."

My third guru in these matters was my father. Along with the keys to the store, he offered me a piece of unexpected advice: "The business of business is to forget business." Although he had never studied Buddhism, my father had a sort of innate Zen about him. Perhaps more from a simple desire for health and peace of mind than for any spiritual motivation, he recognized the challenge of being able to go home and get a good night's sleep, no matter how things were going at the store.

My respect for the Hindu view of life's stages continued to deepen the longer I studied meditation. I observed repeatedly that just going off into seclusion doesn't seem to help anyone too much in the long run. At least in the West, to help us grow into open, compassionate, and wise people, meditation usually needs to be practiced as part of an engaged and active life in our society.

Nonseparation is the bottom line and real challenge of meditation: continually letting go of our boundaries and experiencing everything and everyone as a part of ourselves. The broader we can extend our embrace of nonseparation, the deeper our enlightenment. In a cave, because there is no one, the opportunities are limited. We are limited living in some spiritual community where everyone is quiet and soft and has the same gentle aspirations as ourselves. It seems that my whole generation is arriving at this conclusion. We can best realize the depths of our divinity by exploring the breadth of our humanity in numerous settings.

After a decade at Playmates, I suspected I had learned whatever lessons it held for me and wished to devote my life more completely to the Dharma. At that time, I came across these lines from the Sufi poet, Rumi:

We've given up making a living.
It's all this crazy love poetry now.
It's everywhere—our eyes, our feelings,
our words—all consumed with it.[1]

The poem was a perfect expression of my aspirations to shed mer-   *247*
chant responsibilities. I copied it, folded it, and placed it in a corner of my
altar. Soon, I was freed of the store. My son came forward to continue the
family tradition.

[1] Translated by Coleman Barks

Michael Attie joined his generation's pilgrimage to the East in the 1960s, living and studying in ashrams and Zen monasteries. He owned Playmates of Hollywood for many years, and founded Dharma Banners, a company that produces prayer flags in English. Attie also founded and teaches dharma at the Don't Worry Zendo in Los Angeles. This essay is an excerpt from *Memoirs of a Lingerie Monk,* a book in progress.

Homage! In Jetsunma, union of all the Three Jewels,
I and all beings take refuge. Having aroused the aspiring thought
of enlightenment, may we enter upon the path profound.

The crowns of the *devas* and *asuras* bow to your two lotus feet.
Liberator from poverty, homage to Tara, Mother.

Please Noble Tara, heed me! After all my afflictions, without exception,
are pacified, may the supportive circumstances and fruition
of my hopes be effortlessly and spontaneously achieved.

FROM THE *SADHANA OF TARA, AN OCEAN OF OFFERINGS*
COMPILED BY HIS HOLINESS JIGDAL DAGCHEN SAKYA

❖

HER EMINENCE SAKYA DAGMO KUSHO

Homage to Tara

I WAS BORN IN TIBET, AND AT AN EARLY AGE I WAS INTRODUCED TO TIBETAN Buddhism by my late uncle, His Eminence Deshung Rinpoche. Since then I have lived in three different countries, and I have seen many changes, including the loss of my country to China, man's trip to the moon, the breakup of the mighty Soviet Union, and numerous other seemingly impossible events. However, a constant in my life has been my faith in the Buddha Dharma. It has always been there for me.

There are many Buddhas, Bodhisattvas, and deities in Tibetan Buddhism. My personal deity is Tara, whom I have honored for many years now. Tara is a female Bodhisattva, or enlightened being. I have received initiations, teachings, and oral transmissions on Tara from many learned teachers and finally, on the insistence of my teachers and my husband, His Holiness Dagchen Rinpoche, I began teaching. As one of the few female Tibetan Buddhist teachers, I feel fortunate to be in a position to benefit people from all parts of the world. At the same time, it is a humbling experience to be often referred to as an emanation of Tara. As Buddhists, one of the first things we learn is humility. As the self or the ego is the root of all worldly suffering, it is important to keep the self in check. However, since my students persist in referring to me as an emanation of Tara, I bear the additional responsibility of portraying all her finest qualities.

Initially, I was a little hesitant to teach highly educated students, but I soon realized that I could really reach out to people and benefit them in ways that neither education nor wealth can. What it boils down to is faith. I have seen miracles happen in my lifetime, and faith is definitely a miracle in itself. Many of my students are doctors, alternative medicine practitioners, and healers. They come to see me, receive initiations and teachings, and honor Tara, and I see the reflection of their faith in their work and their relationships with their patients. When they have an understanding of the basic principles of the Buddha's teachings, and with a firmer commitment to the practice of Tara, I have felt the compassion of these healers as they use their special gifts for healing the sick. I have seen women who had problems conceiving be blessed with a baby after practicing Tara. There are mentally troubled people who walk away more relaxed, with a sense of focus as they chant the mantras in praise of Tara. Such miracles don't happen every day in my life, but when they do they give me great joy and satisfaction.

As a female teacher, I feel that women can relate to me directly and personally and that has helped me forge many friendships with some wonderful and compassionate women, who in turn help to promote the message of Tara. As sentient beings we are all dependent on one another. Just as my students depend on me for guidance and solutions, I depend on them to practice patience and compassion. I learn a lot from their lives and experiences, and I put away a piece of them in my heart to remember them and pray for their happiness.

I am the mother of five sons and have seven grandchildren, and I continue to learn something new at every turn. The practice of the Buddha Dharma, and in particular the practice of Tara, has enriched my life, and it is my dearest wish to share this precious feeling with all those who come to me. I learned as a little girl to generate kindness and regard all sentient beings as one's own mother and therefore develop infinite compassion for all beings. I have faith that my students will bring their understanding of kindness and compassion into their homes and bring up their children to be better human beings.

Tara made a pledge to Avalokiteshwara (Buddha of compassion) that she would always take birth in female form until she could remove all beings from the sufferings of *samsara* (the worldly cycle of birth and rebirth). To be born as a human being is precious and to be born as a female is doubly so, for we have the power to give birth and have the patience to bear tremendous pain, which characterizes great strength. I therefore feel very fortunate to be a woman, for we all have a purpose in this world, and I feel close to mine. "May the radiant flower of Tibetan tradition be preserved for the benefit of all beings."

253

Her Eminence Sakya Dagmo Kusho is the founder and teacher of the Mother Tara Sakya Center. Born in Kham, Eastern Tibet, she began her training in Buddhist practice at an early age, as she is the niece of one of the most highly realized Sakya masters of the twentieth century, H.E. Deshung Rinpoche III. When she married H.H. Dagchen Rinpoche, she became Sakya Dagmo (Holy Mother) of the Sakya Khon family, one of Tibet's religious family lineages. She coauthored a book, *Princess in the Land of Snows,* about her life in Tibet and her family's escape over the Himalayas in 1959. Dagmo Kusho has received extensive teachings and empowerments from revered lamas throughout her lifetime.

Namu Dai Busa.
Throw your life into the arms of the Buddha.

SOEN ROSHI

✧

BARBARA PENN

Just This

SOMETIMES CERTAIN WORDS AND CIRCUMSTANCES COME TOGETHER IN SUCH A way that the world loses its grip, a part of the brain slips back, and something inside shifts. In a sense, words fail, but in a wonderful way. They vanish beyond the chained synapses of thoughts in the brain to something deeper, to reveal the message that's always been there: "just this."

One of those circumstances occurred a few months ago in California while I was listening to a Dharma talk by Zen teacher Joko Beck. Joko's words hit me as solidly as a handful of thrown stones, splitting open the shells of memory and meaning inside my head. After years of Zen practice, of hearing certain similar words over and over, somehow this was different.

I asked myself, How come? Why was this different? Was this "feeling" anything I could put into words, and if so, what would they be?

Joko's Dharma talks are always an expression of who she is: a person naturally in her life; there are no edges of personality, and so there is never any strain or reach. Her talks are deceptively simple, as elegant as a mathematical equation, nothing extra. This talk, too, was extraordinarily simple on the surface.

On the surface, the canvas Joko was painting was a picture of Soen Roshi, one of her former teachers. The first brush strokes: "A remarkable teacher; kind, a true monk; completely ordinary in his life, except when you were in his presence and felt the compassion, the true love." Another brush stroke, Soen's vow: *Namu Dai Busa* (Throw your life into the arms of Buddha). He chanted this vow, she said, all the time and in all kinds of places: "Out in the woods on his knees, *Namu Dai Busa;* in a Catholic monastery, on his knees before the image of Christ, *Namu Dai Busa.*" "Always," she said, "the vow pushing his practice." It was with Joko's words, "vow pushing his practice," that the canvas disappeared. I felt the way I sometimes do reading a poem or listening to a symphony. The hairs on the back of my neck stood up as I felt the unspoken frame that held her words.

258

I read once about a man who lived on the edge of a desert. Each day he went out with his broom and attempted to sweep up the desert floor. One day someone came across him, astonished by what he saw, and asked the man, "Why are you sweeping the desert? Don't you see it's useless?" The man answered, "It's an opportunity because it is an impossible task at which to work, exactly as one might meditate or pray."

And so Joko's talk was for me the handle of that broom in my own life. I saw that it's "useless" but that it is okay. Here was Joko, today and every day, always and ceaselessly attempting to find the words, knowing the impossibility of the search. In her attempt, she shows us Soen Roshi, day in and day out, on his knees, bowing humbly. He is not ascending the mountain but coming down it to where his life, and mine, is lived, with "the vow pushing his practice."

Our practice is the ceaseless sweeping of the sand, the endless grains of beliefs, concepts, and thoughts. We continue doing this impossible task because it is the opportunity to see who we really are. We continue doing it, even when the winds kick up and the sand stings and we don't want to do it at all, sensing we will never get it all swept. This is the only vow to take.

Listening to Joko, I remembered many other words. "The still point of the turning world." "Thy will, not mine, be done." Words I loved to play with, spin around in my head, words the truth of which I thought I understood. I recalled the aspirations and the little prayers I'd said over and over through Catholic elementary and high school, the words encircling my brain as stiffly as my uniform blouse collar. The words mixed with the insistent smell of incense and candle smoke and holiness as I repeated over and over silently, "Thy will, not mine, be done." As a schoolgirl, this aspiration and these words were magic, an incantation that I recited not on Mala beads but rosary beads. I felt as I whispered the words that if I said them often enough, fervently enough, then somehow the blazing light of Christ, Wisdom, and Peace would shine down on me, cleansing me, making me free. Even as I said these words, I knew there was a huge gap between this Christ and me.

259

Many years later, I became a Buddhist and took what is known as the precepts, a set of vows. The three pure precepts, "Do not create evil, practice good, actualize good for others," are followed by what are called the ten grave precepts. And now in a small room in California, here was Joko, living the vows. Through her words, Soen was alive—the embodiment of the everyday, actual functioning of the vows. Their meaning was not in the taking of them, nor in their words, or in adding anything extra. They express the simple willingness to keep looking at "just this," to be naturally in whatever our own right life is, nothing big or extraordinary or unattainable. They express our willingness to look at what's happening now, allowing us, as William Blake suggests, to kiss the joy (or sorrow) as it flies by.

Recently I planted a butterfly bush in my tiny garden in North Carolina. It doesn't look like much; certainly it does not have the elegance of rose bushes or azaleas that demand attention with their flood of color and scents. It's a very ordinary bush, except to the butterflies who merge with it, completely losing their own shape, color, and form. Unless you were to shake the bush, the butterflies are indistinguishable from it; they are not separate. But neither is the bush separate from the butterfly. Together, they are an expression of "butterfly bush." Yet the bush is a bush, and the butterfly a butterfly.

The vow is the vow, the practice is the practice, but with the vow pushing our practice—our practice the simple, day-to-day acts, the vow the day-after-day willingness surrounding it—they are the practice-vow, an expression of life, just this, as it is.

Barbara Penn, a Zen student at Zen Center of San Diego, has been meditating for almost twenty years. She is cofounding editor of *Kshanti* literary magazine. She is a published fiction writer, recipient of the Breadloaf and Yaddo fellowships, designs Web pages for businesses and universities, and runs writing workshops. Penn is also a therapist who works with disturbed children, their families, and schools. She hopes to set up a Zen hospice in the future to train at-risk youth as caregivers.

He is the blue bird, he is the green bird with red eyes;
he is the thundercloud, and he is the seasons and the seas.
He has no beginning; he has no end.
He is the source from which the worlds evolve.

FROM THE *UPANISHADS*

JIM RYAN

A New View of Time

I ONCE TOOK A LONG TRAIN RIDE FROM DELHI TO MADRAS; IT WAS SOMETHING like thirty-six hours. We stopped, seemingly for no reason, at a small country junction in the hinterlands of Andhra Pradesh. There was no explanation for the stop and no prediction of when the train would start again. I was anxious and infuriated. I paced up and down the platform asking anyone I could for an explanation, but none was forthcoming. As the hour dragged on to several hours, I was in a state. Suddenly I noticed how the other people on the train were reacting. They had spread out blankets on the platform and they were socializing, smiling and laughing, thoroughly relaxed. They were enjoying this unexpected, unexplained interruption in their journey. I got the feeling from them that if the train never started again it would be okay. This was a new view of time, not one that needs it to be carefully sliced and trimmed, but one that just accepts it, and welcomes its passing through our existence. Rather than trying to control time, the people were delighted to let it control them for however long this train breakdown took. Theirs was an attitude of openness and joyful acceptance of unpredictability; it was an extraordinary bit of wisdom.

I used to go to the large village of Madurai in the south and sit on a big hill called Elephant's Mountain. It was called this because its shape was that of an elephant's head with its long trunk trailing back. The hill was known for being a site where two thousand years ago Jain ascetics would go to do the rite of *Sallekhana,* a rite of starving to death, under-taken to defeat the last of one's *karma* and ensure liberation from birth and rebirth. The stone beds that they had carved and hollows for keeping water were still there. I sat up there, smoked marijuana, and watched the kites float listlessly on the hot wind. I could see the famous temple of Madurai with its towers built in the seventeenth century and looked out in four directions at the very green rice fields filled with field-workers. I could see the bullock carts carrying their burdens to and from Madurai, and the world slowed down. If I forgot about the trucks and automobiles that crept down the ancient thoroughfares in the distance, I felt that I saw the same things that the ancient ascetics did as they lay down to let their lives slip away. The kites held a moment in the air and time stopped. I felt an eternal truth there on Elephant Mountain—that same truth that I found on the train platform. Time leaves endless tracks, but in our true selves we are beyond it, silent witnesses.

I learned another lesson sitting at a local tea stall. People in the West also drink tea or coffee and while away the hours. But an Indian tea stall, or *chai* stall, is a different matter. It seems like a cup of tea lasts *forever.* There is a sense of just being there drinking from an endless cup. People don't read or keep themselves busy in a tea stall. They might idly chat, but mostly they just look at the world as it goes by. There is a sense of an eternal wit-nessing that transcends time.

In India, I learned to give up my Western craving for predictable units of time, even for predictability itself. Waiting for trains; sitting on an ancient hill; drinking a cup of tea: these common experiences have been my *Upanishads.*[1]

---

[1] The *Upanishads* are mystical texts composed in India from 800 to 400 B.C.E., that speak about the unitary nature of ultimate reality. They are central texts that are authoritative for almost all of later Hinduism.

Jim Ryan received a Ph.D. in South Asian Tamil literature from the University of California at Berkeley. His interests are the culture, history, and philosophies of India, specifically the various forms of Hindu *tantra*. He has a secondary interest in Jainism and the historical interplay between the nontheistic philosophical tradi-tions and Hinduism.

We do not listen because our minds are too occupied, and our occupations are petty. Even the mind that is occupied or concerned with the search for God is petty because it is occupied. It is only the mind that is free, quiet, and unoccupied that has bliss, that has infinite space; to such a mind comes that which is eternal.

J. KRISHNAMURTI

MARK ROBERT WALDMAN

I Was a Jewish Atheistic Ministerial Counselor with a Buddhist Practice Who Prayed to God, Went with the Taoist Flow, Embraced Confucian Morals, and Frolicked with a Hindu Goddess or Two

YES, YES, I KNOW—IT'S THE LONGEST TITLE FOR A MINI-MEMOIR THAT'S EVER BEEN penned in English, but I really don't give a damn, for when you've tinkered with as many spiritual disciplines as I have, you can upturn any cart you find even if you accidentally kill a Buddha along the way.

Of course, it's easier if you happen to be born Jewish or semi-Jewish or have a circumcised uncle or two. So what if you drop out of Hebrew school the day after you're Bar Mitzva'd? So what if you take the Talmud to heart and you question the existence of God? So what if you succeed in demolishing the meaning of life? After all, existential angst and agnostic oblivion aren't as bad as they sound. Just head off to a California college or ashram, then cash in those graduation government bonds for a one-way ticket to the East. Any country will do, for with those hippie beads and bushy hair and a girlfriend named Dorothy or Toto or Oz, you'll fit right in as you hitchhike down the yellow brick road of enlightenment. Read a little Kerouac and Castaneda, play the sitar with Ravi Shankar, then chant a few chants in a mosque. Hari Krishna, Hari Rama, Rama Rama, hari-kari.

Well, it doesn't take much acid to see that I was lost, so I packed my bags and cut my hair and headed for the desert to find truth. Instead, I found a couch. What the hell, I thought, so I lay down at a million bucks an hour and channeled Sigmund Freud.

"Say vatever comes to mind, vithout censoring anything at all, you pitifully neurotic soul," he whispered with a sneer.

"But Krishnamurti said I must go deeper if I want to pluck out the roots of my despair." Before poor Siggy could respond, ol' Yackananda butted in, so I just let loose and howled. By god, it was a ride as insane as any cactus juice could produce, and I started shouting about mothers and penises and Oedipal rocks with such fervor and fanaticism and flame that my analyst jumped out of his chair and cheered. Miracle of miracles, he even *talked*, but I never found Jesus or God.

So I quit the couch and headed back East—East L.A., that is—and buried myself in books. From Erich Fromm to Alan Watts, from Suzuki to Kornfield and Grof, I read myself to death, living on a diet of Ram Dass, Haagen-Dazs, and beer. Through the infinite black holes of the mind I pondered my navel and nostrils until I finally came down with a cold. Lying there, prostrate upon my bed, my mind suddenly came to a stop. Finally— *finally*—I was there. Samadhi. Sartre-ori. Ravioli, cream cheese, and bliss. One Big Bang of the brain and the whole damn universe fell into place and I knew, absolutely, positively, beyond the shadow of a Jungian doubt that *this* was all there was.

Enlightenment was mine.

Then the moment passed. I was back in my body, back in L.A., and back to the analyst's couch, this time a born-again therapist peddling *koans* and kreplach to Christians, Kabbalists, and kids. I had insight to sell, and I even slowed down and relaxed, for I had all the time in the world.

To smell the flowers and sage in my yard.

To give my son a small hug.

To kiss my parents before they passed on.

And share a few jokes with my friends.

Especially jokes, because when you're a Jewish atheistic ministerial counselor who consults the *I Ching* while flirting with the goddesses of love, a little Sufi humor is needed to help you stay with the flow. Thank Allah for the wisdom and compassion of the East.

Mark Robert Waldman is a writer, editor, and therapist with a counseling practice in Woodland Hills, California. He is the author and editor of nine books and anthologies including *Love Games, The Art of Staying Together, The Spirit of Writing,* and *Dreamscaping.* He is the founding editor of *Transpersonal Review,* an academic literature review journal covering the fields of psychology and religion.

Whatever you do, make it an offering to me—the food you eat,
the sacrifices you make, the help you give, even your suffering.
In this way, you will be freed from the bondage of *karma*,
from its results both pleasant and painful.

BHAGAVAD GITA

❖

SHIVA REA

Life As Offering

I started reading the *Bhagavad Gita* as an Ashtanga yoga student in Mysore, South India, some ten years ago. The *Gita* captured my imagination and turned my ideas about yoga on their heads. The teachings in the story went straight to my heart like the arrow of Arjuna, the consummate hero and master archer whom we find at the beginning of the *Bhagavad Gita*, uncharacteristically on his knees, shaken to his depths. As he is about to blow the conch to begin the war against his half-brothers the Kauravas who are destroying the earth they unrightfully rule, he becomes paralyzed with fear, doubt, and confusion.

His choice is difficult. How can he act violently against his own blood? Arjuna's dilemma is what makes the *Bhagavad Gita* a universal spiritual classic. Because we have all been in seemingly unsolvable situations, we listen carefully to the seeds of wisdom flowing from Arjuna's chariot driver, who is none other than Krishna, an incarnation of the Divine. His counsel is the opposite of what we might expect from a warrior when the *Bhagavad Gita* was written some two thousand years ago. He gives Arjuna teachings on the all-pervading power of love. He counters our ideas of yoga as a path of withdrawal from the world and defines yoga as "wisdom in action." He speaks of the essential practice of offering, *dana*, which is to surrender attachment to the future and to become fully present and aligned with the Source: "Whatever you do, make it an offering to me—the food you eat, the sacrifices you make, the help you give, even your suffering. In this way, you will be freed from the bondage of *karma,* from its results both pleasant and painful." This passage entered me, and then it seemed wherever I turned all I could see were offerings.

272   In India, the practice of offering, or *puja,* permeates the rhythm of daily life. From morning to night, life is punctuated by the color and vitality of offerings to a myriad of different deities in the form of fragrant flowers, mangoes and bananas, incense, red and orange powders, milk and ghee. When I was studying yoga in Mysore, one of my favorite parts of the day was walking to practice at 4:00 A.M. with only the mothers in the side streets making their morning offerings to the goddess Laxmi. Using rice flour and pigment, every morning women draw a fresh *yantra* to align their homes with the Divine. As the feet of all who enter step on the sacred diagram, it gradually fades, until the next morning when it is created again. Before cooking, bathing, or eating, more *pujas* are offered. Wherever I turned in Mysore, under trees, in shops, in rickshaws and buses, altars to different deities created endless opportunities for remembrance. I loved to stand at a corner where a street-side shrine dedicated to the goddess faced the chaotic flow of traffic. Without fail, all the motorists, whether in car, cycle, or rickshaw, closed their eyes for a moment as they passed, bowing their heads in a gesture of reverence.

Soon, the sun salutations at the beginning of my yoga practice became moving offerings. And I took up Krishna's advice about offering "even your suffering," and offered the intensity of my sensation in deep hip openers and backbends. The offerings of my practice, my bowels and pollution-coping lungs, were humble compared to the man who muttered mantras while pulling a cart huge enough for an ox, or the coal-dark eyes of the hungry child begging on the street. With each of my own offerings, I remembered the big picture and honored the source of the diversity of life. The same energy that makes a tree grow propels me to move and revs the engines of wild rickshaws. The *Gita* opened me to the offerings that permeate Hindu Indian life. Offerings that an outsider might see as empty ritual became for me profound reminders of the underlying source of life.

Still engaged in yoga *sadhana*, I feel like a fish that once swam in the sea and must now learn to breathe in the confined secular space of America. When I returned home to Los Angeles, I found myself looking for shrines on the streets as if they were present but invisible to my eyes. This is not a romantic longing as India is as direct a reality check as one can receive. What I miss are the effects the shrines and altars had on my movement in dance, in yoga, in the world.

My practice is more internal now. I see the messes my two-year-old son makes as offerings to creativity, and the surrendering of harsh words as an offering to love. When teaching yoga, I find I have infinitely more stamina and grace when I offer my energy to the well-being of my students. I offer the content of my mind, giving my judgments to the fires of compassion and offering my resistance as kindling to the flames.

Shiva Rea was given her name by her father, which led her to the study of yoga at the age of fourteen. She practices and teaches *vinyasa* (flow) yoga, integrating alignment and intuition, strength and fluidity, meditation and wisdom in action. She is based in Santa Monica, California, and leads adventure retreats worldwide. Her Web site is www.yogadventures.com.

There is a Light that shines beyond all things on earth, beyond us all,
beyond the heavens, beyond the highest, the very highest heavens.
This is the Light that shines in our heart.

CHANDOGYA UPANISHAD

❖

Thine own consciousness, shining, void, and inseparable from
the Great Body of Radiance, hath no birth, nor death,
and is the Immutable Boundless Light.

PADMASAMBHAVA,
THE TIBETAN BOOK OF THE DEAD

❖

MATTHEW COLEMAN

Composting Light

THIS MORNING ON MY WAY TO MY MEDITATION CUSHION, IN THE WOODS BEHIND our house, I pass the compost pile once again. But this time the bright orange flowers of the volunteer squash catch my eye and I stop and gaze in wonder at this vigorous, huge plant.

A single seed, a tough seed that withstood the trials of this compost pile, somehow managed to sprout. It survived the winter freeze, the intense burning heat that good compost generates, the hungry bugs, maybe a hidden nest of mice and marauding, digging dogs. This one seed has lived and grown and survived. The warmth generated when the light touches the earth activated the latent life in this one seed. The genetic map unfolds; a sprout pushes up to the sun while a tiny rootlet pushes down into the earth. The rootlet gathers nourishment from the water, the soil, and the molecules of air that have seeped down into the pile. The upward-growing sprout transforms out into a leaf and then another and another. Alive, these leaves transform sunlight into more life, more of itself. It is all light. Even the very dark earth that these plants grow from is nothing but light. Light from above, light from below. Have you ever seen molten lava roll brightly down a mountainside? This fiery burning heat is thick liquid light. We call the light from below hell; we call the light from above heaven. Strange, isn't it? It's only a matter of direction.

Looking at this plant, I see magnificent green leaves, big bright orange flowers rising up as offerings to the butterfly and the bumblebee, and to me as I pause for a moment in reverent revelation.

Tiny little tendrils curl around and grab on and hold upright and pull this squash plant upward, toward more and more light. Being human, I have a need and a love of light: the sun on my back, the light reflected off rippling waters, the reflections in my mind of the infinite images in this beautiful world. I don't know where exactly this ancient cycle of life and light began. I do know that this terrifying primal light, from below and from above, is the fuel that keeps the engines burning.

There is also a primal light I have seen, a light that manifests in me. It comes from very deep within, beyond my mind, deeper even than the bottom of my heart. It seems from somewhere else entirely. It is so bright I shy away; so vast, I am awed by its force. It exposes me, humbles me. I tremble, I prostrate myself before this light in me. The source of me, the end of me, the all of me.

I am nothing more than a fragile-skinned leaf transforming light to life. Changing light to laughter, light to pain, light to love and caring. Is there anything more to life than this transformation, this play, this dance of atoms and molecules? The compost pile at my feet reflects the light, pushes out the leaf, ever-transforming light to life.

Matthew Coleman is a student and practitioner of the Kagu lineage of Tibetan Buddhism. His main teachers are Kalu Rinpoche and Lama Drupgyu. Coleman has taught Buddhist meditation for fifteen years. He lives with his wife on Salt Spring Island, British Columbia, Canada, where he writes, gardens, kayaks, and plays with his grandchildren.

La Noche Oscura

ST. JOHN OF THE CROSS

En una noche oscura,
con ansias en amores inflamada,
¡oh dichosa ventura!
salí, sin ser notada,
estando ya mi casa sosegada.

A oscuras, y segura,
por la secreta escala disfrazada,
¡oh dichosa ventura!
a oscuras y en celada,
estando ya mi casa sosegada.

En la noche dichosa,
en secreto, que nadie me veía
ni yo miraba cosa,
sin otra luz y guía
sino la que en el corazón ardía.

Aquesta me guiaba
más cierto que la luz del mediodía,
adonde me esperaba
quien yo bien me sabía,
en parte donde nadie parecía.

¡Oh noche, que guiaste,
oh noche amable más que la alborada:
oh noche, que juntaste
Amado con amada,
amada en el Amado transformada!

The Dark Night

TRANSLATED BY SHINZEN YOUNG

On a dark night,
On fire with longing for love,
Oh happy venture!
I left, unseen,
My house being still . . . at last.

In darkness, and safe,
By the secret stairway, in disguise,
Oh happy venture!
In darkness and concealed,
My house being still . . . at last.

Into the happy night,
In secret, for no one saw me
And neither did I see anything,
Without light or guide,
Other than that which burned in my heart.

And this guided me,
More surely than the light of noon,
To where He awaited
One well known to me
In a place where no one would appear.

O night that guides!
O night more lovely than the light of dawn!
O night that unites
The Lover with the beloved,
And transforms the lover into the Beloved!

En mi pecho florido,
que entero para él solo se guardaba,
allí quedó dormido
y yo le regalaba,
y el ventalle de cedros aire daba.

El aire de la almena,
cuando yo sus cabellos esparcía,
con su mano serena
en mi cuello hería,
y todos mis sentidos suspendía.

Quedéme y olvidéme,
el rostro recliné sobre el Amado;
cesó todo, y dejéme,
dejando mi cuidado
entre las azucenas olvidado.

On my flowering breast,
Which I reserved entirely for Him alone,
There He dwelt and slept
And I caressed Him,
And the cedars fanned us with their breeze.

The breeze blew over the castle wall and
As I ran my fingers through His hair,
With His gentle hand
He pinched my neck,
And suspended all my senses.

Thus I stayed, and forgot myself,
Resting my face upon the Beloved;
Everything stopped, and I was set free,
Leaving my care behind
Forgotten, among the lilies.

SHINZEN YOUNG

O Night That Unites:
A Personal Appreciation of St. John of the Cross

THE MEDIEVAL CHRISTIANS HAD A WORD FOR IT—*COINCIDENTIA OPPOSITORUM*—
the unification of opposites. For me the *Noche* of St. John of the Cross rep-
resents not one but many such unifications. For most of my life I have been
a teacher of Buddhist meditation. My approach is "user friendly" but at the
same time "industrial strength." I fully intend for students to reach at least
the initial stages of classical mystical experience. In my tradition, this
comes about through experiencing ordinary events with radical attentive-
ness and openness—so radical that the sensual domain melts into vibrating
space. Eventually even those vibrations die away. Die away into what? This
is the point that is so difficult to convey. They die away into a special kind
of nothing, a "full" nothing that is rich and deeply fulfilling.

Each of the world's traditions has a technical term for this most special nothing. To the Buddhist it is *shunyata;* to the Christian, *nihil per excel-
lentiam.* In the Jewish tradition, they say *ayn;* in the Islamic, *fana'.* Taoists
call it *Wu,* and some Native Americans refer to the empty space between
the sweat lodge's four direction stones.

People are often put off by such negative language, all this talk of
"emptiness" and "no self." Does the *nihil* of the mystic really differ from
the *nihil* of the nihilist? Yes. Because the *path* to the void is different, the

experience of it is different, and radically so! It is a cessation that contains within it the cumulative riches of the entire sensed world. *Todo y nada,* the ultimate *coincidentia oppositorum.*

Read *La Noche Oscura* carefully. On one level it is a richly sensual, almost pornographic account of a young girl's nocturnal romantic adventure.

282

> *The breeze blew over the castle wall and*
> *As I ran my fingers through his hair,*
> *With his gentle hand he pinched my neck . . .*

But at the same time it vividly conveys the vacuous and impersonal nature of *direct* encounters with the Divine.

> *In darkness, and safe . . . without light or guide . . . in a place where no*
> *one would appear . . . everything stopped . . .*

St. John was one of the most hard-core celibate renunciates in the history of Christianity. His practice of self-denial and consensual pain actually frightened his fellow monks. How extraordinary that such a person could portray the sensuality of love with such appreciation.

> *On my flowering breast,*
> *Which I reserved entirely for Him alone,*
> *There he dwelt, and slept*
> *And I caressed him . . .*

Actually it makes sense. Why practice self-denial or self-torture? There are many pathological reasons but only a few healthy ones. Skillful austerity purifies the sense gates by breaking down the viscosity in their flow. This purification reduces suffering, but it also elevates the satisfaction derived from the senses. The way to gauge the effect of your asceticism is not how much you suffer but how much richer and more fulfilling your sensual life becomes. Another unification of seeming opposites.

La Noche Oscura moves me because it so brilliantly portrays the simultaneous richness and vacuity that characterizes the day-to-day experience of a true mystic; the "oneness of Bliss and Void" as the Tibetans put it.

I was originally trained as an academic, and I still have a great love for study and research. Although known for his poems, St. John was also a well-educated scholastic in the Catholic intellectual tradition. Many people read *La Noche Oscura* and are touched by the level of feeling. But what most people don't know is that every phrase in the poem relates to some specific aspect of contemplative technology or Christian doctrine. St. John intended to write a detailed prose commentary on the poem explaining its subtle intellectual content, but he did not live long enough to complete it. His goal was to unite the affective energy of a lyrical poem with the intellectual impact of a carefully reasoned essay—another integration of worlds.

I grew up Jewish in Los Angeles during the 1950s. My early relationship to the Christian world around me was one of fear and loathing. When I began Buddhist practice in Japan in the late 1960s, I was amazed to find many Catholic priests and nuns participating in Buddhist retreats there. Through contact with these people, I came to realize that the experiences I was having as a Buddhist meditator had parallels in Christianity, that indeed there is a universal core of meditative and mystical experience shared by all cultures and times. Understanding this universality has allowed me to find a harmony among my Jewish background, my Buddhist training, and the Christian milieu in which I live.

Think of how different our worlds are, San Juan de la Cruz and I. He: A sixteenth-century Roman Catholic priest writing for the very Inquisition that expelled my ancestors from Spain. Me: A twenty-first-century Jewish Buddhist technorationalist. Yet, reading *La Noche Oscura*, his greatest poem, I can honestly say, "Yes, I understand what your life was ultimately about. That's where I live too."

Shinzen Young, a native of Los Angeles, became fascinated with Asian culture at an early age, learning Chinese and Japanese while still in his teens. In 1968, he entered a doctoral program in Buddhist studies at the University of Wisconsin. Three years later he was ordained as a Buddhist monk at Mount Koya, Japan. He has worked at the Princeton Biofeedback Institute and taught Asian philosophy at Chapman College and mathematics and physics at Ernest Holmes College. He serves as translator for Joshu Sasaki Roshi at Mount Baldy Zen Center. Shinzen has been conducting meditation retreats throughout North America for more than twenty years. His Web site is www.shinzen.org.

There is no need for temples
No need for complicated philosophy
Our heart is our temple
The philosophy is kindness.

HIS HOLINESS THE FOURTEENTH DALAI LAMA

PHYLLIS WATTS

The Soft Underbelly of Life

MUCH OF MY LIFE HAS BEEN SPENT IN MY MIND. THE WORLD OF IDEAS, OF CONCEPTS and constructs, of analysis and synthesis has always been as real to me as the material world. In many ways, it has been more real. After all, I have reasoned, the idea of a table existed before the table itself.

My curiosity and need for a conceptual framework for life have compelled me to study philosophy, psychology, and the religions of the world. Ideas have always ignited my mind and led me on a pursuit of truth. In my personal and professional communities I am known for my discursive treatises on subjects so disparate as to be comical. Yet when I look closely at each of these, they have at their core an argument for a whole other way of being. In truth, what holds me, soothes me, comforts me, and terrifies me in its sometimes motherly, sometimes banshee arms, is the purity of lived experience. Just this moment. Right now. I'll take experiences of any kind, but those that especially hold me are imbued with kindness and sincerity and an openness to the many flowerings of humanity around us, whether they be radiant or repugnant.

Early on in my sojourn on this wily planet I came to understand that the world of experience was little respected by people with power and smarts. In the way only a clever girl from the working class can, I wanted to be accepted by them. I truly admired the weird, disembodied, analytic respectability that is garnered by mannered circles. But I genuinely could not understand the way these same circles virulently rejected experience as a legitimate way of knowing about life. In our polite and tony discussions, I would argue, conceptually of course, for this other way of knowing. And, again and again, I was withered by the gentle dismissal of what I knew to be true.

288

Their arguments were inspired by their fear, though I didn't know it then. They were afraid of the oozy, roiling underwater currents of life, afraid of diving deep into their own murky interior worlds or knowing about what was right across the tracks from their own neighborhoods. They preferred instead the pristine perspective of deep-sea fishing; discussing and analyzing from the safe distance of knowing *about* things versus knowing them through direct experience. Experience involves the body and the heart. It is messy and unruly and associated with all things unrefined, irrational, earthy, mysterious, feminine. Experience is the soft underbelly of life. It is where all things are understood and encoded, even when we deny it.

So while I actually practiced deep-sea diving, plunging, sometimes dangerously, into the mysterious realms of life, I pretended to go deep-sea fishing and stay above it all. I would grab some tiny morsel of experience to immediately be brought up into the rarified air of reason for relentless dissection. I became good at passing. I became so good, in fact, that I forgot I was just pretending. But there always moved in me a vague uneasiness, a knowledge of what was really so for me, and what I really believed life was about.

And then, many years ago, through the oddest set of circumstances, I found myself invited to an international conference in Costa Rica by a group I had never heard of and haven't heard from since. At the conference, among other renowned dignitaries, was His Holiness the Dalai Lama. He spoke about seeking the true meaning of peace. I was undone.

I'm not completely sure what it was about him or his words that so moved me. The best way I can describe it is that I deeply identified with his expression of what was important and real. He spoke about being straight with ourselves, being kind to others, and being responsible for how we tread upon this planet. It did not escape me that he is a learned man, a man of true intellect and reason. His mind is brilliant. Yet he made it clear that the mind is secondary to the heart. Simple human kindness and compassion for others are the basis of life. They cannot merely be discussed and argued. They are not an idealized construct. They are practical and must be lived.

289

I felt I had come home to my heart, and this experience is repeated each time I see him, read his words, or hear him speak. He advocates and, I believe, lives what I have known to be true from the time I was a sprig of a girl. Through genuine kindness and compassion for others, practiced in the moment, we weave the fabric of our days. At the same time we mend the tattered fibers of suffering and indignity that each of us has endured.

Today the intellectual and experiential parts of my soul are starting to form a holy alliance. Experience leads the way through its devotion to sincerity and kindness. Reason delicately teases apart, then synthesizes all that experience has gathered.

Phyllis Watts, Ph.D., has studied philosophy, psychology, and the religions of the world for over three decades. She is the president of Wild Swan Resources, a consultancy devoted to helping organizations and their leaders cultivate wisdom in business and life. Additionally, she is a licensed psychologist, dancer, and avid volunteer.

Vairochana, pure and clear Dharmakáya Buddha;
Lochana, full and complete Sambhogakáya Buddha;
Shákyamuni, infinitely varied Nirmánakáya Buddha;
Maitreya, Buddha still to be born;
All Buddhas everywhere, past, present, future;
Mahayana Lotus of the Subtle Law Sutra;
Mañjushrí great wisdom Bodhisattva;
Samantabhadra, great action Bodhisattva;
Avalokiteshvara, great compassion Bodhisattva;
All venerated Bodhisattavas, Mahásattvas,
The great Prajñá Páramitá.

THE TEN NAMES OF THE BUDDHA
A ZEN MEALTIME *SUTRA*

❁

SUSAN SUNTREE

The Green Bean *Sutra*

In 1984, WHEN I PARTICIPATED IN MY FIRST FIVE-DAY *SESSHIN* (RETREAT) AT RING of Bone Zendo in northern California, I was amazed, confused, and, most important, alert, as I am when I travel alone through new territory. As a brand-new Zen student, experiencing the activities of daily life as formalized practice deeply affected me. From one moment to the next, I had no idea what would happen or how to behave.

Orioki, the ritualized mealtime practices and chants, for example, left me fumbling with cloths, bowls, and chopsticks. I felt like a beginner in dancing school, tripping and waving my hands while all the others gracefully, fluidly, moved through the meal from one gesture to the next until the final folding of the napkin and the tying of the knot. According to the custom at Ring of Bone, when the servers bearing trays of food enter the Zendo, all chant "The Ten Names of the Buddha":

> *Vairochana, pure and clear Dharmakáya Buddha;*
> *Lochana, full and complete Sambhogakáya Buddha;*
> *Shakyamuni, infinitely varied Nirmánakáya Buddha;*
> *Maitreya, Buddha still to be born;*
> *All Buddhas everywhere, past, present, future;*
> *Mahayana Lotus of the Subtle Law Sutra;*
> *Mañjushrí great wisdom Bodhisattva;*

Samantabhadra, great action Bodhisattva;
Avalokiteshvara, great compassion Bodhisattva;
All venerated Bodhisattavas, Mahásattvas,
The great Prajñá Páramitá.[1]

Meal after meal we recited while I dithered, finally settled, and ate my food.

During this *sesshin,* as is the Zen practice, all participants spend part of each day supporting the needs of the retreat community. For my work practice I was assigned to the food-chopping crew. In the white summer light, we choppers stood at long, outdoor tables facing piles of the day's vegetables and fruits to be prepared for the coming meals. Beyond our station, a straw-gold meadow spread to the bordering pine and madrone forest. Dry heat, even by midmorning, radiated from dusty green and yellow surfaces. Insects purred in the grasses, softening the thumps and staccato beats of our chopping.

I had come to the *sesshin* laden with grief and worry about a dissolving marriage. And as the marriage had fragmented, so had my sense of self. My anxieties wavered like sunlight on the stone pathways. One day we were presented with a mountainous heap of green beans to chop. One by one I took the curling, tender pods, laid each one out on my board, cut off its stem and blossom ends, and chopped it into 1-inch-long pieces. I had to look carefully at the shape of each bean and eventually small groups of beans, as I became more adept with my knife. Each bean spoke to me about its nature:

Pure and clear green bean;
Full and complete green bean;
Infinitely varied green bean;
Still to be born green bean;
Past, present, future green bean;
Lotus of the subtle law green bean;
Great wisdom green bean;
Great action green bean;

Great compassion green bean;
All venerated green beans.

The mealtime *sutra* (scripture) repeated in my mind over and over as I chopped. Each bean was a glorious sacrifice; the basket of beans was an infinite lineage of Buddhas passing through my hands to become our lunch, offering immediate and practical nourishment.

I stopped chopping for a moment and examined the nearby forest. Some trees had trunks that bent at odd angles to reach the sunlight, and others were stunted by the canopy shading the places where they were rooted, and others grew tall and mostly straight. All were uniquely formed by their neighbors, shaping and reshaping one another: The forest grew in dynamic perfection. Who would criticize a bean for its peculiar curl or a tree for its particular trunk, even the most stunted tree in the grove?

Then I looked at my hands. I didn't see the knife; I saw my arms and followed their trail to my body. I stopped still as this moment engraved itself onto my memory. Even now I can see the luminous meadow, the dark green fringe of trees, the beans curling together on the wooden chopping table, and my own body: pure and clear, full and complete, infinitely varied. But the image blanked out and I stood, once again, feeling anxious and incomplete.

I rebelled against this continuum, this wholeness made up of many precious, unpredictable moments because obviously it included me. When I looked around at my fellow choppers, I knew it included them, too—each one lifting and lowering a knife, making a meal with energy and attention as well as with fruits, flowers, stalks, roots, seeds, and leaves. And I knew that if it included them, all hungry humanity was included, and the whole hungry universe: gullet, tongue, fangs, and lips. I wouldn't accept the other people or myself. We stood apart from nature. We were too flawed, too greedy, too cruel, and too wrenchingly harmful to ever be accounted for by such a generous description. I went back to my chopping, but the green beans wouldn't lie still. "The Ten Names of the Buddha," replaced by the beans, have stayed with me for nearly two decades.

295

In 1996, at dawn on a gray July morning, I picked up a bullhorn and explained to long lines of trapped rush-hour motorists why helicopters, fire trucks, and the police had converged at Jefferson and Lincoln Boulevards, near Los Angeles International Airport. We were standing in the heart of the 1,087-acre Ballona Wetlands, an important stopover for birds on the severely threatened Pacific Flyway and the location of significant Native American archeological sites. Three people, one of whom is blind, their wrists handcuffed inside steel pipes, had locked themselves onto bulldozers that were being used to destroy the wetlands.

Participating in this action catalyzed my commitment to help save the last open spaces in Los Angeles, a city not normally associated with either open space or environmental activism. But these efforts are often fraught with dangers, sometimes involving face-to-face conflicts with corporate security squads and the police, and sometimes emotional conflicts within environmental groups. When my heart pounds and my mouth goes dry with fear, in my endeavor to stay open hearted, I remember the basket of beans and the forest and whisper the Green Bean *Sutra*. It prompts me to recall the multiple ways we opponents and compatriots influence and shape one another. As I walk at the wetlands, I remember, too, that the birds, the sedges, and the moist sea air all participate in the common shaping. Each encounter is pure and clear, full and complete, infinitely varied.

When I stand ready at the chopping table, hand, knife, beans, trees, and troupe of choppers infused with the morning light, I am less likely to retreat into flurries of anxiety, anger, and confusion. Especially if I have wandered away downhearted or discouraged, I recite the Green Bean *Sutra* as a song of recognition, of praise, and as a reminder to lighten up and get back to the table.

---

[1] The full mealtime ceremony can be found in Robert Aitken's *Encouraging Word: Zen Buddhist Teachings for Western Students* (New York: Pantheon Books, 1993).

Susan Suntree, editor of this anthology, incorporates her Zen practice and environmental activism into her writings and performances about contemporary culture. She has a son and a daughter and lives in Los Angeles.

We venerate the Three Treasures
And are thankful for this meal
The work of many people
And the sharing of other forms of life.

ZEN BUDDHIST GRACE

GARY SNYDER

Grace

THERE IS A VERSE CHANTED BY ZEN BUDDHISTS CALLED THE "FOUR GREAT VOWS." The first line goes: "Sentient beings are numberless. I vow to save them." *Shujō muhen seigando.* It's a bit daunting to announce this intention—aloud— to the universe daily. This vow stalked me for several years and finally pounced: I realized that I had vowed to let the sentient beings save *me*. In a similar way, the precept against taking life, against causing harm, doesn't stop in the negative. It is urging us to *give* life, to *undo* harm.

Those who attain some ultimate understanding of these things are called "Buddhas," which means "awakened ones." The word is connected to the English verb "to bud." I once wrote a little parable:

Who the Buddhas Are

All the beings of the universe are already realized. That is, with the exception of one or two beings. In those rare cases the cities, villages, meadows, and forests, with all their birds, flowers, animals, rivers, trees, and humans, that surround such a person, all collaborate to educate, serve, challenge, and instruct such a one, until that person also becomes a New Beginner Enlightened Being. Recently realized beings are enthusiastic to teach and train and start schools and practices. Being able to do this develops their confidence and insight up to the point that they are fully ready to join the seamless world of interdependent play. Such new enlightened beginners are called Buddhas and they like to say things like, "I am enlightened together with the whole universe" and so forth.

BOAT IN A STORM, 1987

Good luck! one might say. The test of the pudding is in the *eating*. It narrows down to a look at the conduct that is entwined with food. At mealtime (seated on the floor in lines) the Zen monks chant:

> *Porridge is effective in ten ways*
> *To aid the student of Zen*
> *No limit to the good result*
> *Consummating eternal happiness*

and

> *Oh, all you demons and spirits*
> *We now offer this food to you*
> *May all of you everywhere*
> *Share it with us together*

and

> *We wash our bowls in this water*
> *It has the flavor of ambrosial dew*
> *We offer it to all demons and spirits*
> *May all be filled and satisfied*
> Om makula sai svaha

And several other verses. These superstitious-sounding old ritual formulas are never mentioned in lectures, but they are at the heart of the teaching. Their import is older than Buddhism or any of the world religions. They are part of the first and last practice of the wild: *Grace*.

Everyone who ever lived took the lives of other animals, pulled plants, plucked fruit, and ate. Primary people have had their own ways of trying to understand the precept of nonharming. They knew that taking life required gratitude and care. There is no death that is not somebody's food, no life that is not somebody's death. Some would take this as a sign that the universe is fundamentally flawed. This leads to a disgust with self, with humanity, and with nature. Otherworldly philosophies end up doing more damage to the planet (and human psyches) than the pain and suffering that is in the existential conditions they seek to transcend.

The archaic religion is to kill god and eat him. Or her. The shimmering food chain, the food web, is the scary, beautiful condition of the biosphere. Subsistence people live without excuses. The blood is on your own hands as you divide the liver from the gallbladder. You have watched the color fade on the glimmer of the trout. A subsistence economy is a sacramental economy because it has faced up to one of the critical problems of life and death: the taking of life for food. Contemporary people do not need to hunt, many cannot even afford meat, and in the developed world the variety of foods available to us make the avoidance of meat an easy choice. Forests in the tropics are cut to make pasture to raise beef for the American market. Our distance from the source of our food enables us to be superficially more comfortable, and distinctly more ignorant.

Eating is a sacrament. The grace we say clears our hearts and guides the children and welcomes the guest, all at the same time. We look at eggs, apples, and stew. They are evidence of plentitude, excess, a great reproductive exuberance. Millions of grains of grass seed that will become rice or flour, millions of codfish fry that will never, and *must* never, grow to maturity. Innumerable little seeds are sacrifices to the food chain. A parsnip in the ground is a marvel of living chemistry, making sugars and flavors from the earth, air, water. And if we do eat meat it is the life, the bounce, the swish, of a great alert being with keen ears and lovely eyes, with foursquare feet and a huge beating heart that we eat—let us not deceive ourselves.

We too will be offerings—we are all edible. And if we are not devoured quickly, we are big enough (like the old down trees) to provide a long, slow meal to the smaller critters. Whale carcasses that sink several miles deep in the ocean feed organisms in the dark for fifteen years.

(It seems to take about two thousand years to exhaust the nutrients in a high civilization.)

At our house we say a Buddhist grace:

We venerate the Three Treasures (teachers, the wild, and friends)
And are thankful for this meal
The work of many people
And the sharing of other forms of life.

Anyone can use a grace from their own tradition (and really give it meaning), or make up their own. Saying some sort of grace is never inappropriate, and speeches and announcements can be tacked onto it. It is a plain, ordinary, old-fashioned little thing to do that connects us with all our ancestors.

A monk asked Dong-shan: "Is there a practice for people to follow?"
Dong-shan answered: "When you become a real person, there is such
a practice."

Sarvamangalam, Good Luck to All.

Gary Snyder teaches literature and wilderness thought at the University of California at Davis and lives with his family on San Juan Ridge in the Sierra foothills. Between working as a logger, a trail-crew member, and a seaman on a Pacific tanker, he studied Asian languages at Berkeley (1953–1956), was involved with the Beat movement, and lived in Japan (1956–1964). He later studied Rinzai Zen Buddhism in Japan for twelve years. He has won numerous literary prizes, including a Guggenheim fellowship (1968) and the Pulitzer Prize (1975).

Compassion should be directed impartially toward all sentient beings
without discriminating between those who are friends and those who are
strangers. With this compassion constantly in mind, every positive act, even
the offering of a single flower or the recitation of a single mantra, we should
do with the wish that it may benefit all living creatures without exception.

All sentient beings are the same in wishing to be happy and not to suffer.

The great difference between myself and others is in numbers: there is only
one of me, but countless others. So, my happiness and my suffering are
completely insignificant compared to the happiness and suffering of infinite
other beings. What truly matters is whether other beings are happy or
suffering. This is the basis of the mind determined to attain enlightenment.

We should wish others to be happy rather than ourselves, and we should
especially wish happiness for those whom we perceive as enemies and
those who treat us badly. Otherwise, what is the use of compassion?

DILGO KHYENTSE RINPOCHE

MATTHIEU RICARD

The Practice of Compassion

DILGO KHYENTSE RINPOCHE, MY TEACHER, WAS BORN IN 1910 IN EASTERN TIBET. Even as a little boy, Rinpoche manifested a strong desire to devote himself entirely to the religious life. Before his main teacher passed away, Khyentse Rinpoche promised him that he would unstintingly teach whoever asked him for Dharma. So to first prepare himself—he was only fifteen when his teacher died—he spent most of the next thirteen years in silent retreat. In remote hermitages and caves deep in the steep wilderness of wooded hills near his birthplace in the valley of Denkhok, he constantly meditated on love, compassion, and the wish to bring all sentient beings to freedom and enlightenment.

After all these years spent in the mountains, Khyentse Rinpoche told his second teacher that he wished to spend the rest of his life in strict solitary meditation retreat. "The time has come for you to teach and transmit to others all the countless precious teachings you have received," was his teacher's answer. Until his death in 1991, Khyentse Rinpoche worked for the benefit of beings with tireless energy.

Khyentse Rinpoche's achievements in different fields each seem more than enough to have filled a whole lifetime: twenty years or so spent in retreat; an astonishing depth and breadth of teaching, taking up at least several hours a day for over half a century; twenty-five large volumes of written works; numerous major projects to preserve and disseminate Buddhist thought, tradition, and culture. With all these undertakings, Khyentse Rinpoche tirelessly gave form to his lifelong dedication to Buddhism.

Everywhere he went, Rinpoche taught, comforted, and inspired all who came to see him. The teaching of Buddhism is not based on some exotic, inaccessible philosophy. It deals with the most basic mechanisms of happiness and suffering and shows how true and lasting happiness can only come from inner peace. Such peace can only be reached by cultivating unselfishness, love, and compassion and by eliminating egotism, hatred, and greed.

Profoundly gentle and patient though he was, Khyentse Rinpoche's presence, his vastness of mind and powerful physical appearance, inspired awe and respect. With close disciples and attendants he could be very strict, for he knew that a good disciple "grows strong under strong discipline." He never spoke harshly to visitors or those not committed to him, but with his own disciples he was uncompromising in making sure that they never got away with shabby behavior, words, and thoughts. To those living near him it was also somehow obvious that he could see clearly through any pretense or hypocrisy. Although the Buddhist teachings point out that there is no better witness than one's own mind, his loving yet formidable presence had a powerful influence on his disciples and ensured that their minds did not wander.

Many great men and women, apart from their particular genius in science or the arts, are not necessarily good human beings. Khyentse Rinpoche was someone whose greatness was totally in accord with the teachings he professed. However unfathomable the depth and breadth of his mind might seem, from an ordinary point of view, he was an extraordinarily good human being. Those who lived near him, even for ten or fifteen years, say that they never witnessed a single word or deed of his that harmed anyone. His only concern was the present and ultimate benefit of others. Here was a living example of what lay at the end of the spiritual path and the greatest possible inspiration for anyone thinking of setting out on the journey to enlightenment.

Matthieu Ricard, a former biology researcher, is a writer and photojournalist who has been a Buddhist monk for over twenty years. He is an interpreter for the Dalai Lama and served as Khyentse Rinpoche's assistant for the last fourteen years of Rinpoche's life. Ricard has translated numerous works about Buddhism.

You know, if you can't say all this stuff simple enough for me to understand, then that means one of two things: Either what you're saying is bullshit, or else you don't understand it yourself.

TED

BO LOZOFF

Ted

IN 1967, MY WIFE SITA AND I STRUCK UP A FRIENDSHIP WITH A 300-POUND hillbilly, ex-con truck driver named Ted. Sita and I were just beginning to get involved in the civil rights movement around the University of Florida. Ted had spent nine years in prison in his home state of Nebraska, and then migrated to Florida with his wife and four kids to start a new life. He was working on a rural construction crew light-years away from the politics of campus life. But one day, while driving a black coworker home from work, Ted was pulled over by a county sheriff's deputy for no other reason than having his coworker in the car. The deputy told Ted, "We don't mix white folks and niggers around here," and the deputy then proceeded toward the passenger side of the car to "teach that boy a lesson for riding with a white man." Ted followed him around the car and knocked him out cold as the deputy attempted to shove him aside. When the student activist community in Gainesville read in the local papers about Ted sitting in jail for reacting to the deputy's racism, Ted became an instant local celebrity. His bail was paid, liberal lawyers rushed to his defense, and a few of us were intrigued enough to meet his wife and four kids and get to know them.

Living in dire poverty, Ted and his family were among the most naturally sincere and honest people we have ever met. They were just good, decent folks with tremendous capability and common sense. Sita and I stayed with them off and on, and Elsie taught Sita about farm cooking and canning and all sorts of things that proved valuable when we later became rural people ourselves. In 1969, Sita and I drifted away and went through profound changes, immersing ourselves in meditation and yoga and Eastern spiritual teachings.

310

Several years passed before we saw Ted and Elsie again. In 1974, they came to visit us at the North Carolina ashram where we were living. My wild hair and beard were gone. I no longer owned a gun, let alone carried one, as I had when we were militant activists. Now, Sita and I wore white clothes and sported long prayer beads. We had become vegetarians and oh so gentle. Ted, always direct, asked us to explain what the hell we were into. He thought maybe we had been taken in by some sort of cult. I responded with eloquent, long-winded truths about spirituality and illusion and Dharma and meditation and transformation and the *chakras* and breathing and energy and . . . you get the point. Ted looked straight into my eyes the whole time, and when I finished, he spit out a little chewing tobacco and said one thing that has shaped my life's work ever since: "You know, Bo, if you can't say all this stuff simple enough for me to understand, then that means one of two things: Either what you're saying is bullshit, or else you don't understand it yourself." That was one of the truest and deepest things anyone has ever taught me.

Ted has long since, as they would say in Tibet, "departed for more fortunate rebirths," but that one piece of unpretentious wisdom lives on in my lectures, workshops, books, and in my life itself. If I can't say it simply, either it's not true, or I don't get it. My first book, *We're All Doing Time,* took seven years to write for that sole reason. Each time I would compile four hundred or so pages, I would begin reading it through Ted's eyes and realize that once again, I had turned the world's classic spiritual teachings into so many complex words and concepts. As this was before the computer age, there was no easy editing. I tossed the whole thing into the wastebasket and began again on a blank first page. That happened at least a half-dozen times before I was able to write from the simplest depths of my heart rather than from my mind.

My lifestyle has changed over time. My spiritual practice has changed over time. But Ted's always in the back of my mind saying, "Remember, spiritual practice should be helping you to become simpler, not more complex; more caring, not less; more resilient and good humored and adaptable, not less." During times when I am at odds with my whole environment, I step back and take a bigger, simpler look once again. It helps me to use the image of a rope. When a rope is knotted up in complicated ways, it may take a lot of effort and various skills to untie it. To me, spiritual practices are merely various ways of unknotting the rope. Ironically, many of us use those very same practices to tie even more knots in our ropes—juggling our schedules endlessly to make time for practice, knocking ourselves out to attend every lecture or retreat, adopting various esoteric fashions or rituals that make us less adaptable or tolerant to environments other than our own. So I frequently remember dear old Ted, and I try to keep the essence of my spiritual life and practices very simple.

Since the time of Ted's death, I have led approximately six hundred prison workshops around the United States and in several other countries, as far away as India. Never once have I prepared anything to say. I just look out on those faces and see my old friend waiting for me to tell him about the deepest sacred teachings that have meant so much to me. I know that every great tradition emphasizes heart over head, devotion over knowledge, faith over intellect. I know that if I embody the teachings in my own affection and respect for the people in front of me, they can understand the Great Traditions. On the way into San Quentin once, a woman from the Buddhist community asked me what I was going to talk about in my presentation. I replied, "When you go to a friend's house for the evening, do you prepare what you are going to say? I'm getting together with friends tonight. That's all." Friends, of course, talk about what's important to them. What's important to me is the spiritual journey and the Great Teachings, so any conversation with me will undoubtedly include stories and insights and practices that I cherish. Ted's one-line piece of advice nearly thirty years ago has enabled me to communicate from my heart rather than my head. I will be forever grateful.

Bo Lozoff and his wife, Sita, are directors of the Human Kindness Foundation in Durham, North Carolina. They have worked with prisoners for over twenty-five years. Lozoff's first book, *We're All Doing Time*, has been translated into several languages. His other books include *Lineage and Other Stories, Just Another Spiritual Book, Deep & Simple: A Spiritual Path for Modern Times*, and *It's a Meaningful Life: It Just Takes Practice.* In 1994, Lozoff and Sita received the Temple Award for Creative Altruism. In 1999, Lozoff was awarded an honorary doctorate from the Chicago Theological Seminary.

312

UNIVERSAL DECLARATION OF HUMAN RIGHTS

On December 10, 1948, the General Assembly of the United Nations adopted the Universal Declaration of Human Rights, the full text of which appears below. All member countries were asked to publicize the text of the Declaration and "to cause it to be disseminated, displayed, read, and expounded principally in schools and other educational institutions, without distinction based on the political status of countries or territories."

In accordance with that call to conscience and consciousness, please copy and disseminate the following document.

PREAMBLE
Whereas recognition of the inherent dignity and of the equal and inalienable rights of all members of the human family is the foundation of freedom, justice and peace in the world,

Whereas disregard and contempt for human rights have resulted in barbarous acts which have outraged the conscience of mankind, and the advent of a world in which human beings shall enjoy freedom of speech and belief and freedom from fear and want has been proclaimed as the highest aspiration of the common people,

Whereas it is essential, if man is not to be compelled to have recourse, as a last resort, to rebellion against tyranny and oppression, that human rights should be protected by the rule of law,

Whereas it is essential to promote the development of friendly relations between nations,

314

Whereas the peoples of the United Nations have in the Charter reaffirmed their faith in fundamental human rights, in the dignity and worth of the human person and in the equal rights of men and women and have determined to promote social progress and better standards of life in larger freedom,

Whereas Member States have pledged themselves to achieve, in cooperation with the United Nations, the promotion of universal respect for and observance of human rights and fundamental freedoms,

Whereas a common understanding of these rights and freedoms is of the greatest importance for the full realization of this pledge,

Now, Therefore,

THE GENERAL ASSEMBLY

proclaims

THIS UNIVERSAL DECLARATION OF HUMAN RIGHTS as a common standard of achievement for all peoples and all nations, to the end that every individual and every organ of society, keeping this Declaration constantly in mind, shall strive by teaching and education to promote respect for these rights and freedoms and by progressive measures, national and international, to secure their universal and effective recognition and observance, both among the peoples of Member States themselves and among the peoples of territories under their jurisdiction.

Article 1.

All human beings are born free and equal in dignity and rights. They are endowed with reason and conscience and should act toward one another in a spirit of brotherhood.

Article 2.

Everyone is entitled to all the rights and freedoms set forth in this Declaration, without distinction of any kind, such as race, colour, sex, language, religion, political or other opinion, national or social origin, property, birth or other status. Furthermore, no distinction shall be made on the basis of the political, jurisdictional or international status of the country or territory to which a person belongs, whether it be independent, trust, non-self-governing or under any other limitation of sovereignty.

Article 3.

Everyone has the right to life, liberty and security of person.

Article 4.

No one shall be held in slavery or servitude; slavery and the slave trade shall be prohibited in all their forms.

Article 5.

No one shall be subjected to torture or to cruel, inhuman or degrading treatment or punishment.

Article 6.

Everyone has the right to recognition everywhere as a person before the law.

Article 7.

All are equal before the law and are entitled without any discrimination to equal protection of the law. All are entitled to equal protection against any discrimination in violation of this Declaration and against any incitement to such discrimination.

Article 8.

Everyone has the right to an effective remedy by the competent national tribunals for acts violating the fundamental rights granted him by the constitution or by law.

Article 9.

No one shall be subjected to arbitrary arrest, detention or exile.

Article 10.

Everyone is entitled in full equality to a fair and public hearing by an independent and impartial tribunal, in the determination of his rights and obligations and of any criminal charge against him.

Article 11.

1. Everyone charged with a penal offense has the right to be presumed innocent until proved guilty according to law in a public trial at which he has had all the guarantees necessary for his defense.

2. No one shall be held guilty of any penal offense on account of any act or omission which did not constitute a penal offense, under national or international law, at the time when it was committed nor shall a heavier penalty be imposed than the one that was applicable at the time the penal offense was committed.

Article 12.

No one shall be subjected to arbitrary interference with his privacy, family, home or correspondence, or to attacks upon his honour and reputation. Everyone has the right to the protection of the law against such interference or attacks.

Article 13.

1. Everyone has the right to freedom of movement and residence within the borders of each state.

2. Everyone has the right to leave any country, including his own, and to return to his country.

Article 14.

1. Everyone has the right to seek and to enjoy in other countries asylum from persecution.

2. This right may not be invoked in the case of prosecutions genuinely arising from non-political crimes or from acts contrary to the purposes and principles of the United Nations.

Article 15.

1. Everyone has the right to a nationality.

2. No one shall be arbitrarily deprived of his nationality nor denied the right to change his nationality.

Article 16.

1. Men and women of full age, without any limitation due to race, nationality or religion, have the right to marry and to found a family. They are entitled to equal rights as to marriage, during marriage, and at its dissolution.

2. Marriage shall be entered into only with the free and full consent of the intending spouses.

3. The family is the natural and fundamental group unit of society and is entitled to protection by society and the State.

Article 17.

1. Everyone has the right to own property alone as well as in association with others.

2. No one shall be arbitrarily deprived of his property.

Article 18.

Everyone has the right to freedom of thought, conscience and religion; this right includes freedom to change his religion or belief, and freedom, either alone or in community with others and in public or private, to manifest his religion or belief in teaching, practice, worship and observance.

Article 19.

Everyone has the right to freedom of opinion and expression; this right includes freedom to hold opinions without interference and to seek, receive and impart information and ideas through any media and regardless of frontiers.

318

Article 20.

1. Everyone has the right to freedom of peaceful assembly and association.

2. No one may be compelled to belong to an association.

Article 21.

1. Everyone has the right to take part in the government of his country, directly or through freely chosen representatives.

2. Everyone has the right of equal access to public service in his country.

3. The will of the people shall be the basis of the authority of government; this will shall be expressed in periodic and genuine elections which shall be by universal and equal suffrage and shall be held by secret vote or by equivalent free voting procedures.

Article 22.

Everyone, as a member of society, has the right to social security and is entitled to realization, through national effort and international cooperation and in accordance with the organization and resources of each State, of the economic, social and cultural rights indispensable for his dignity and the free development of his personality.

Article 23.

1. Everyone has the right to work, to free choice of employment, to just and favorable conditions of work, and to protection against unemployment.

2. Everyone, without any discrimination, has the right to equal pay for equal work.

3. Everyone who works has the right to just and favorable remuneration ensuring for himself and his family an existence worthy of human dignity, and supplemented, if necessary, by other means of social protection.

4. Everyone has the right to form and to join trade unions for the protection of his interests.

Article 24.
Everyone has the right to rest and leisure, including reasonable limitation of working hours and periodic holidays with pay.

Article 25.
1. Everyone has the right to a standard of living adequate for the health and well-being of himself and of his family, including food, clothing, housing and medical care and necessary social services, and the right to security in the event of unemployment, sickness, disability, widowhood, old age or other lack of livelihood in circumstances beyond his control.

2. Motherhood and childhood are entitled to special care and assistance. All children, whether born in or out of wedlock, shall enjoy the same social protection.

Article 26.
1. Everyone has the right to education. Education shall be free, at least in the elementary and fundamental stages. Elementary education shall be compulsory. Technical and professional education shall be made generally available and higher education shall be equally accessible to all on the basis of merit.

2. Education shall be directed to the full development of the human personality and to the strengthening of respect for human rights and fundamental freedoms. It shall promote understanding, tolerance and friendship among all nations, racial or religious groups, and shall further the activities of the United Nations for the maintenance of peace.

3. Parents have a prior right to choose the kind of education that shall be given to their children.

Article 27.

1. Everyone has the right freely to participate in the cultural life of the community, to enjoy the arts and to share in scientific advancement and its benefits.

2. Everyone has the right to the protection of the moral and material interests resulting from any scientific, literary or artistic production of which he is the author.

Article 28.

Everyone is entitled to a social and international order in which the rights and freedoms set forth in this Declaration can be fully realized.

Article 29.

1. Everyone has duties to the community in which alone the free and full development of his personality is possible.

2. In the exercise of his rights and freedoms, everyone shall be subject only to such limitations as are determined by law solely for the purpose of securing due recognition and respect for the rights and freedoms of others and of meeting the just requirements of morality, public order and the general welfare in a democratic society.

3. These rights and freedoms may in no case be exercised contrary to the purposes and principles of the United Nations.

Article 30.

Nothing in this Declaration may be interpreted as implying for any State, group, or person any right to engage in any activity or to perform any act aimed at the destruction of any of the rights and freedoms set forth herein.

PERMISSIONS

Grateful acknowledgment is made to the following:

John Adams, "Lost in Movement, Found in Stillness" © 2001 by John Adams.
Robert Aitken, "Carvers" © 2001 by Robert Aitken.
Jill Ansell, "Asanga and the B Yard" © 2001 by Jill Ansell.
Michael Attie, "Memoirs of a Lingerie Monk" © 2001 by Michael Attie.
Michael Barnard, "The Infinite Well" © 2001 by Michael Barnard.
Joko Beck, "The Key" © 2001 by Joko Beck.
Jacquie Bellon, "You're Preapproved—Accept Today" © 2001 by Jacquie Bellon.
Grace Brumett, "Gone Beyond: A Question of Letting Go" © 2001 by Grace Brumett.
Melody Ermachild Chavis, "Going to Prison" © 2001 by Melody Ermachild Chavis.
Pema Chödrön, "Finding Our Own True Nature." Excerpted from *The Wisdom of No Escape* © 1991 by Pema Chödrön. Reprinted by arrangement with Shambhala Publications, Inc., Boston, MA. www.shambhala.com.
Cheri Clampett, "A Knowing Beyond Words" © 2001 by Cheri Clampett.
Bob Cohen, "Saint or Sinner?" © 2001 by Bob Cohen.
Matthew Coleman, "Composting Light" © 2001 by Matthew Coleman.
Baba Hari Dass, "God Is Peace." Excerpted from *For the Love of God* © 1997, edited by Richard Carlson and Benjamin Shield. Reprinted with permission of New World Library, Novato, CA 94949. www.newworldlibrary.com.
Norman Fischer, "My Mother." Excerpted from *Jerusalem Moonlight: An American Zen Teacher Walks the Path of His Ancestors* © 1995 by Norman Fischer. Clear Glass Press, San Francisco. Reprinted by permission of the author.
Geshe Tsultim Gyeltsen, "The Buddha's Great Heart" © 2001 by Geshe Tsultim Gyeltsen.

ABOUT THE EDITOR

Susan Suntree is a writer, performer, and teacher whose work investigates the dynamics of science, art, and spiritual philosophies as they engage contemporary life. She has presented her poetry and performances nationally and internationally and has published books of poetry, biography, and translation, as well as essays, reviews, and book chapters. Her recent one-woman performance, *Sacred Sites/Los Angeles*, explores the prehistory and sacred geography of Los Angeles, where she lives. She is the founder of FrogWorks, an ecopolitical street theater troupe, and codirector of Earth Water Air Los Angeles, a giant puppet trek across the city connecting endangered open spaces. An environmental activist and a long-time Zen student, she currently teaches at East Los Angeles College.

INDEX

A
❀

acceptance
  of time passing, 263–64
  of what is, 53, 123, 157–59
activism, 167–68, 309, 310
  environmental, 44, 296
  mindfulness and, 81–85
altars, 30, 196, 272, 273
  meditating at, 195, 196
anger, 83, 153, 154, 211
animals, compassion for, 70–71, 90–91,
  135, 193–94
arrogance, 34–35, 174, 175, 176
art, and life, 115–16
aspirations, higher, within everyone,
  130
attachments to world, letting go of,
  122–23
awareness
  concern for world and, 81
  interreligious, 84
  too busy for, 97
  turning inward, 6

B
❀

bamboo flute. See *shakuhachi*
beauty, 115, 116–17, 223–27
  primeval, 117
  response of heart to, 115
birth, 253
body
  mindfullness of, 141, 147
  separation of soul from, at death,
  211–12
boundaries, letting go of, 246
brain, 257, 264
breathing
  counting breaths in, 148, 164
  mindfulness of, 148–49
  pleasure of, 149
business, 245–46
busyness
  of daily life, 97, 165–68, 190, 245–46
  of the mind, 35, 148, 165–166, 167,
  190
butterfly bush, 259

C
❋

calm mind, 29
  meditation and, 39, 57, 189
  yoga and, 25
cancer
  death and dying and, 63–66, 211–12, 215–19
  P'howa prayer and, 212
  yoga and, 141
caregiving, 51–52, 63–65
Carvers metaphor, 17–18
centeredness, yoga and, 22
childhood, wisdom of, 3–4
commitment, 205–6
  escaping, 206–7
  as frightening, 206
  marriage and, 206–7
  to practice Buddhist precepts, 258–59
  to self, 207
communication
  compassion and, 90
  with spirits, 5
community, wisdom and compassion
    and, 84
compassion, 3–4, 70–71, 77, 89, 90–91, 135–36, 196, 252, 253, 289
  for animals, 70–71, 90–91, 135
  communication and, 90
  community and, 84
  insight into, 90
  vegetarianism and, 135
consciousness
  creative, 190
  deeper level of, 190
  of dying persons, 64–65
  everyday, 57
  during meditation, 57
  state of, effect on experience and
    knowledge, 188–89
  transference of, at time of death, 211–12, 218–19
  yoga and, 139, 140–41
control, letting go of need for, 60
counseling, spiritual, 211–12, 216–18
cranes
  origami, 5
  sounds of, 103

criticism, 69–70
  mind busy with, 35
  versus negativity, 81

D
❋

daily life
  busyness of, 165–68, 190, 245–46
  compassion in, 89–90, 91
  Green Bean *Sutra*, 293–96
  in India, 263–64, 272
  mindfulness in, 40
  priorities in, 84
  values in, 85
dance, 115–17
death and dying, 29, 30, 64–65, 145, 158, 211–12
  cancer and, 63–66, 211–12, 215–19
  food and, 301
  letting go, 215–19
  prayer to help with, 211–12
  sudden, 212
  transference of consciousness and, 211–12, 216
  yoga and, 139–40
distraction, mindfulness as antidote
    to, 39
diversity, 3–4

E
❋

eating, 300–301. *See also* mealtime
  as sacrament, 301–2
ego
  keeping in check, 251
  letting go of, 122
  ehipassiko, 51–53
empathy, lack of, 202
emptiness, 65, 219, 281–82
  of mystical experience, 281–82
  terms of various religions for, 281
energy, 195, 196
engagement, constructive, 81, 82–83
  defined, 81
  without anger, 83–84
enjoyment of life, 59–60
enlightenment, 268, 299–300
  nonseparation and, 246

environmental activism, 44, 296
experience
  versus reading, 14–15
  reason and, 289
  world of, 287, 288

F
❋
faith, 202–3
  as miracle, 252
feminine characteristics, 237–42, 238,
  253, 288
flute, bamboo. See *shakuhachi*
focusing, 48
foolish friends, 34
freedom, 205, 206
  to make a commitment, 207
  marriage and, 206

G
❋
generosity, 70–71
God, 121–23
grace, at mealtime, 301–2
Green Bean *Sutra*, 293 96
grief, 29, 30, 63–66, 211–12

H
❋
happiness, 69, 149
  mindfulness and, 146–48
Hare Krishna Movement, 127–30
harmony, 183
healing, 6
  elements in us, being in touch with,
    149
  faith and, 252
  love and, 4
  mindfulness and, 40
  yoga and, 139
health
  mental clarity and, 189
  yoga and, 139–41
Healy, Jack, 76
heart
  learning to look into, 97
  mind as secondary to, 289
  playing *shakuhachi* from, 109, 111

response to beauty, 115
  working from, 48
heart-knowing, versus intellect, 25
hiding, 96–97
  coming out of, 97–98
  no real place for, 97
  in work, 97
human rights, 76–77
  Universal Declaration of Human
    Rights, 313–20
humility, 237, 238, 251

I
❋
illness, 51–53, 63–66. *See also* cancer
  yoga and, 139–40
insights
  brain and, 257, 268
  readiness for, 190
  into true compassion, 90
  yoga and, 22–23, 140–41, 141
intellect
  versus heart-knowing, 25
  versus resolve, 35
interconnectedness, 194

J
❋
jealousy, 69–70
joy, 45, 147, 148, 206

K
❋
kindness, 34
knowledge
  letting go of need for, 60
  from soul versus from books, 25
  state of consciousness and, 188–89
Kuan Yin (goddess of love and mercy),
  195

L
❋
Lao-tzu, 181–83, 237–39
leaders, Lao-tzu on, 182
learning, constant, 35
letting go, 215–19
  of boundaries, 246

life
  conceptual framework for, 287
  enjoyment of, 59–60
  investigating joys and sufferings of,
    51–53
  light and, 278
  in present, stepping into, 51–53
  stages of, 245, 246
  as work of art, 116–17
life, purpose of, 6
light, primal, 277–78
liking/disliking, giving up, 10, 14
living without leaving tracks, 142
loss, 29, 30, 211–12
  of mother, 63–66
love, 30, 46, 89, 153–54
  as basis for action, 35
  death and, 219
  of God, 34, 121
  goddess of (Kuan Yin), 195
  healing and, 4
  of lover, 33
  meaning of, 33–34
  prayer and, 196

M

male characteristics, 238
marriage, 206–7
martial arts
  playing, 59–60
mealtime
  chants and rituals, 293–95, 300
  grace at, 301–2
meat-eating, 301
meditation, 12, 39–40, 51, 258. See also
    mindfulness
  concern for world and, 81
  consciousness during, 57
  hiding from self in, 97
  as learning to look into own, 96
  mindfulness and, 39–40
  oneness as goal of, 244
  purpose of, 40
  suizen (blowing meditation), 101–5
  Taoist, 57
  Transcendental Meditation, 187–90
  transcending during, 188–90
  yoga and, 24, 140–41

mental clarity
  health and, 189
  meditation and, 189
mercy, 196
  goddess of (Kuan Yin), 195
mind
  busyness of, 35, 148, 165–66, 167,
    190
  clear, 188–89
  peaceful, 123
  quieting noise in, 190
  as secondary to heart, 289
  states of, 153–54
  subduing, 69
  transforming into vehicle of love, 91
mindfulness, 39–40, 145–49
  as antidote to distraction, 39
  of breathing, 148–49
  constructive engagement and, 81–85
  functions of, 39–40
  happiness and, 146–48
  integrating with everyday life, 40
  meditation and, 40
  practicing, 40
  remembering to practice, 40
moment, present. See present moment,
    living in
Mother, Divine, 237–42
mothers, 33, 35, 51–52, 63–65, 76,
    157–58, 252
motivation, and awareness of
    suffering, 83–84
music, 109–11, 174–75, 223–27
  bamboo flute, 101–5, 109–11
  Western and Japanese traditional,
    101, 104, 109–11
mystical experience, terms for, 281

N

nature, 277–78
  beauty of, 223–27
  divinity in, 5
negativity, 69–70, 153–54
  versus criticism, 81
nonseparation, 246
nonviolence, constructive, function of,
    82

O

oneness, 282
  as goal of meditation, 244
optimism, 76

P

pain, 206
pain, awareness of lack of, as peace,
  147
patience, 25
peace
  inner, God as, 121–23
  mindfulness and, 146–48
  in present moment, 146–48
  walking for, 168
  yoga and, 25
P'howa prayer, 211–12
physical needs, 44–45
play, 59–60
politics, spirituality and, 81
pollution, protesting, 44
possessions, letting go of, 122–23
practice, spiritual, 173–74. *See also*
    meditation
  about finding own true nature, 173,
    175
  Buddhist vow, 258–59
  Chinese martial arts and, 59–60
  purpose of, 97, 258–59
  questions asked in, 96, 98
  stability in, 60
prayer, 4, 196, 258–59
  to help dying leave the body, 211–12
present moment, living in, 29, 51–53,
    145–49
  yoga and, 231–33
present moment, peace in, 146–47
priorities, of daily life, 84
prisons, working in, 9–14, 89–90
purpose of life, 6

Q

qigong, 57
questioning, 97, 98
quiet, 24, 25

R

reading, versus experience, 24–25
real life, 25
  versus books, 24–25
  as only teacher, 29
receptivity, 238, 239
relationships
  escape from, 206, 207
  versus marriage, 206
Remprasad, 237, 240–42
responsibilities
  fulfilling, 35
responsibility, universal, 76, 77
revelations, yoga and, 22–23
Rinpoche, Khyentse, 305–8
Roosevelt, Eleanor, 76, 77

S

St. John of the Cross, 281–83
sculptors, knowledge of, 17–18
search, spiritual, 5, 75–76, 96–98, 127–30
seeking, 245–46
  understanding, 96–98
self
  authentic, 17–18, 146, 175, 177, 216,
    264
  Green Bean Sutra and, 294–95
  hiding from, 97
  knowledge of, and commitment, 206
  lack of commitment to, 207
  shakuhachi as projection of, 104, 105
  working with, to find own true
    nature, 175
self-denial, 282
selfishness, 84
selflessness, 238
seriousness, 59, 60
service, life of, 239
Shabkar, life of, 133–36
shakuhachi (bamboo flute), 101–5,
    109–10, 111, 223–27
  identifying with sound of, 105, 104
  as mirror of player's soul, 104, 110,
    111
  relating to, 111
sight, 147

silence, 24
  inner, 190
simplicity, 241, 310–11
sinners, 127
sleep, 44–45, 246
smiling, 146, 148, 149
soul, transition at time of dying,
    211–12
sounds, 102–3, 104–5
  of bamboo flute, meditation
    through, 102–5
spirituality, and politics, 81
spiritual nature of reality, 189
success in life, 35
suffering, 63–65, 158, 207, 272
  awareness of, and motivation, 83–84
  no-gap intimacy with, 51–53
support of community, 84

T

Taoism, 57
Tao Te Ching, 181–83, 237–39
teacher and student, relationship
    between, 102–3
thought, stopping, and yoga, 23
Tibetan Buddhism, 75, 175–76
time, 47
  accepting passing of, 263–64, 268
  importance of, 24
  Indian view of, 263–64
transcendence, not becoming obsessed
    by, 239
Transcendental Meditation, 187–90
transformation
  into Buddha, 195
  deeper level of consciousness and,
    141
  deep level of compassion and, 91–92

U

understanding
  hiding from, 96
  seeking, 96
United Nations
  Universal Declaration of Human
    Rights, 76–77, 313–20

V

values, in daily life, 85
vegetarianism, 135, 301
violence, 82, 153, 202
visions, 133
vows, Buddhist, 258–59, 299

W

waiting for God, 24
Watts, Alan, 75–76
wholeness, 5
wisdom
  of childhood, 3–4
  community and, 84
  seeking, 95–96
women, 39, 253
work, hiding in, 97
world, attachments to, 122–23
worrying, 148
  stopping, 10, 12, 14, 148–49

Y

yoga, 139–41, 271–73
  approaching study of, 24–25
  Ashtanga Vinyasa, 21–25
  benefits to, 22
  healing and, 140–41
  insights and, 140–41
  living in moment and, 231–32
  meditation and, 24
  thoughts and, 23